BELMONT UNIVERSITY LIBRARY
BELMONT UNIVERSITY
1900 BELMONT BLVD.
NASHVILLE, TN 37212

Lois E. Passi, LCSW

A Guide to Creative Group Programming in the Psychiatric Day Hospital

Pre-publication
REVIEW

"**T**his is a well-written, well-organized book that will be of great use to students, new graduates, and seasoned clinicians. It is easy to follow and gives excellent realistic suggestions not only for day hospital treatment but inpatient units as well. As a licensed clinical social worker with ten years in the field, I learned a great deal from this book and plan to utilize the exercises immediately."

Jennifer Victoria Underwood, MSW
Licensed Clinical Social Worker,
Charter Behavioral Health System

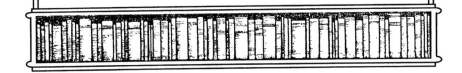

NOTES FOR PROFESSIONAL LIBRARIANS AND LIBRARY USERS

This is an original book title published by The Haworth Press, Inc. Unless otherwise noted in specific chapters with attribution, materials in this book have not been previously published elsewhere in any format or language.

CONSERVATION AND PRESERVATION NOTES

All books published by The Haworth Press, Inc. and its imprints are printed on certified ph neutral, acid free book grade paper. This paper meets the minimum requirements of American National Standard for Information Sciences–Permanence of Paper for Printed Material, ANSI Z39.48-1984.

A Guide to Creative Group Programming in the Psychiatric Day Hospital

HAWORTH SOCIAL WORK IN HEALTH CARE
Gary Rosenberg and Andrew Weissman
Editors

A Guide to Creative Group Programming in the Psychiatric Day Hospital by Lois E. Passi

A Guide to Creative Group Programming in the Psychiatric Day Hospital

Lois E. Passi, LCSW

The Haworth Press
New York • London

© 1998 by The Haworth Press, Inc. All rights reserved. No part of this work may be reproduced or utilized in any form or by any means, electronic or mechanical, including photocopying, microfilm and recording, or by any information storage and retrieval system, without permission in writing from the publisher. Printed in the United States of America.

The Haworth Press, Inc., 10 Alice Street, Binghamton, NY 13904-1580

Cover design by Marylouise E. Doyle.

Library of Congress Cataloging-in-Publication Data

Passi, Lois E.
  A guide to creative group programming in the psychiatric day hospital / Lois E. Passi.
      p.   cm.
  Includes bibliographical references and index.
  ISBN 0-7890-0406-2 (alk. paper).
  1. Psychiatric day treatment—Activity programs. I. Title.
RC439.2.P37 1998
616.89'165—dc21   97-43560
                                                                                                                  CIP

200873
BELMONT UNIVERSITY LIBRARY

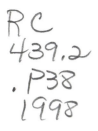

RC
439.2
. P38
1998

ABB-9692

This book is dedicated to Phil.
May the one true Therapist hold you in His arms
and grant you eternal peace.

ABOUT THE AUTHOR

Lois E. Passi, LCSW, is a clinician with University Behavioral Health Care in Piscataway, New Jersey. She is also a certified group psychotherapist with the National Registry of group psychotherapists in New York City. Passi designed and implemented the first clinical program for the Adult Acute Day Hospital of the University of Medicine and Dentistry in Piscataway. In addition, she works extensively with couples as a certified imago relationship therapist.

CONTENTS

Acknowledgments

I would like to thank those who were a part of making this book a reality. Thanks are due to Lenore Baeli-Wang who edited the book and Marc Klein who provided legal advice. Santiago Asuro translated Spanish passages, and Cindy McCoy, LCSW; Sallye Poff, LCSW; and Joseph Reina, MHS, read and critiqued the manuscript.

I also wish to acknowledge my colleagues at University of Medicine and Dentistry of New Jersey–Community Mental Health Center at Piscataway. First, without the staff of the Adult Acute Day Hospital there would be no Day Hospital into which I could bring these groups: Philippe Khouri, MD; Andrea Carsen, RN; Joseph Reina, MHS; Gregory Jones, MHS; Kathryn Popino; Marilyn Blacher-Reich, LCSW, CEAP; and Marcia Clever, MD. Second, my thanks to other colleagues at the Community Mental Health Center who participate in the running of the Day Hospital: Susan Darien, LCSW; Cindy McCoy, LCSW; Sergio Levi-Minzi, MD; Heidi Chihab, RN; and Ernestine Green, RN. Third, I would like to express special thanks to Frank Jones, MD, for his support while I was writing this book.

I am deeply grateful to Vikas Passi for his tremendous support and encouragement.

My greatest thanks by far are due the patients, for they have been my best teachers. When I was called for a job interview with the Day Hospital I was at a low point in my career. I was even considering changing careers. I accepted my new job with a sense of mission and possibility for the patients and for the field. I had no idea what potential existed for my personal growth, nor did I realize that the patients would be the key to that growth. In the beginning, I saw myself as their teacher and guide. Before too long I came to realize that we are mutual teachers and guides of one another.

The patients are always teaching me to be courageous in the face of terrible circumstances. They show me the extraordinary value of life by fighting daily for their lives. They warn me of the immeasurable loss when life is lived in despair. They remind me to be grateful for a life without mental illness.

The patients are not people with diagnoses; neither are they diagnostic categories. They are not schizophrenics, addicts, depressives. They are extraordinary human beings who are learning to live with schizophrenia, addiction, depression. Those illnesses are the circumstances with which they are forced to live—dire circumstances. Yet there is something precious beyond those circumstances that we all possess, something that remains invisible unless we are committed to seeing it. It is inexpressible. Whatever it is, it is that with which I interact daily.

The patients have taught me that the essence of life is in the struggle to live fully, in the lessons learned along the way. In that they have been, and continue to be, my faithful companions. Along the course of my journey, each of these companions has left me a bigger person than I was before I met them. I hope that I have been able to do the same for them.

The Groups in Alphabetical Order

Chapter 1

How to Use This Book

This book was written for clinicians, especially those clinicians charged with designing a clinical program for a day hospital. It is therefore not a book about basic skills in group psychotherapy or other clinical skills. There are plenty of books written on these topics. It is assumed by this writer that the reader possesses basic clinical skills, especially in the area of group psychotherapy. The recent graduate receiving ongoing supervision will be able to utilize this book as well as the experienced clinician.

This book offers ideas for themes and outlines for creative groups that address these themes. Very little is said about process. The group outlines are the skeleton, while the process is the flesh of the group. I provide the skeleton. You provide the flesh.

This chapter begins with a discussion of the *modalities* utilized in this book. These include the use of movie clips, written exercises, oral exercises, therapeutic games, role-play, homework assignments, and what I call the "use of metaphor." Each chapter of the book discusses the *therapeutic themes* addressed in the groups, which include relapse prevention, goal setting and support, cognitive restructuring, activities of daily living, social skills, socialization, self-esteem, affective issues, motivation, and exercise. I also discuss ideas for starting and ending the day. Later in the book I discuss versatility; that is, taking a group outline and adapting it in various ways to fit the needs of the group with which you are working at a specific time.

You should feel free to use these groups as they are presented in the book *or* to alter them in a way that suits you. My only request is that you clearly state, when presenting the group to others, whether you are using my group or your own version. You may also find that you want to invent your own groups. This is ideal since every program is different. If you learn enough from this book to create your own program without using any of the groups outlined in the book, that is fine. The goal is for you to design a top-quality clinical day hospital program. I place particular emphasis on this because the groups I invented were for use with a psychiatric population participating in a short-term day hospital program. The population I had in mind included people with psychotic disorders, affective disorders, and personality disorders. There are many populations I did not have in mind when I was writing, including recovering addicts, Alzheimer's patients, and young children. So the motto for you is "adapt and invent."

A NOTE ABOUT CREATIVITY

Some of you may be saying, "I'm not the creative type. I can't do this." Plenty of people have said this to me. I, therefore, want to offer some encouragement regarding creativity.

First, view everything in your life as potential teaching material for the day hospital. When you go to a movie, be aware of themes and clips that might illuminate issues germane to patients. When you read stories, consider what might be useful. For example, I read the *Mahabharata,* a Hindu epic which includes the famed "Bhagavad Gita." While I was reading the *Mahabharata* for my own personal pleasure, I kept the day hospital in the back of my mind in order to easily recognize useful material for the program. For example, there is a story in it about a king who is addicted to gambling and gambles away his entire kingdom in one day. I thought that the story power- fully illustrated the first of the twelve steps of AA: "We admitted that we were powerless over alcohol (or any addictive substance) and that our lives had become unmanageable." I read the story (after editing out parts of it) to a group for dually diagnosed patients.

Second, ask others for ideas. Most people will tell you about a therapeutic game they played in a workshop or something they heard a colleague do. Their ideas will be the groundwork for your own ideas.

Third, relax. Don't try to force anything. Ideas will naturally come to you. The more you try to force them, the more blocked you will be. When I try to force something, I am never creative. Then, when I'm lying in bed, something just appears in my mind.

Remember to always keep the therapeutic theme central, not the modality. The modality *serves* the therapeutic theme. The milieu *serves* the therapeutic purpose. In other words, you don't want to say, "What kind of group can I make from this movie?" You want to say, "What can I use to discuss the theme of decreasing isolation? Are there any movies that will help me with this?" I can't emphasize this point enough. Many people are pressured to come up with a group. They have some materials (perhaps some art materials or an article) and they ask themselves, "What can I do with this?" This is the avenue for designing a group that serves the clinician's needs, not the patients' needs. It would be better to simply have an open discussion about a topic that is salient for the group than to force a theme from some movie or art material.

STANDARD ACTIVITIES

With some exception, I decided not to discuss standard activities. By standard activities I mean those activities that are often utilized in day hospitals or inpatient units for groups. For example, while I offer a brief discussion about how to view exercise groups from a therapeutic context, I do not discuss specific types of exercise activities. Most programs have equipment for basketball, volleyball, whiffleball, and so forth. I also say nothing about arts and crafts, a frequent activity of inpatient and day hospital programs. Most programs also offer standard vocational groups, which include didactic groups about resume writing, interview skills, vocational goal setting, and so on. Other groups not discussed in this book include the standard, open-forum group psychotherapy, recovery groups for dually diagnosed patients that focus on the twelve-step program, medication education groups, and groups focused on other health concerns, such as safe sex and nutrition. My aim in writing this book is to provide clinicians with creative possibilities beyond the standard groups that are usually offered.

MODALITIES

Earlier I alluded to two different ways of categorizing the groups: by modality and by therapeutic theme. Modality refers to the nature of the milieu itself—to the materials and modes of expression that are used. Using movie clips as a catalyst for discussion is an example of one modality. The movie clips can be used to address a wide variety of therapeutic themes, such as isolation, relapse prevention, and so on.

None of these modalities is unique. Many people have used movie clips to ignite discussions or illuminate themes. Oral and written exercises are certainly not new. Therapeutic games and role-play have been used for years. What I offer in this book is a way of putting these modalities together to create a high-quality day hospital program.

One important aspect of all of these modalities is that they allow you to create a program with very little money. They also allow programming with a minimum of staff and space. It is assumed that many people operate with these restrictions, hence they were kept in mind when designing groups.

Written Exercises

Written exercises help patients to organize and articulate their thoughts about a particular issue. They also provide the patient with something tangible to take home and to refer to in the future. This is especially important because many patients have poor concentration and memory skills. Anything that can be put down on paper has a better chance of being retrieved for future use. Additionally, patients may not be ready to really dig in and do the work on a particular topic when you see them; however, they might be ready to look more closely at that topic six months later. If they can refer to old notes, worksheets, etc., all the better.

Some examples of written exercises offered in this book include Hospitalization Review, The Size of the World, certain parts of the Creating the Support Team series, and Mountain Exercise.

Keep several things in mind about written exercises. First of all, be mindful of people who do not comprehend the written word very well, whether it is because of a language barrier, poor education, or poor intellectual functioning. It may be useful to translate your written exercises into Spanish and any other language you think may be spoken with some frequency by patients in your unit (this is true of all reading material as well). When designing written material, keep the language simple.

You should also be mindful of the person with physical problems who may have difficulty with a writing exercise. For example, cogentin, a frequently prescribed drug that helps to mitigate the side effects of some neuroleptics, causes blurred vision. Lithium as well as other drugs sometimes cause hand tremors, making it difficult for patients to write.

In addition, psychotic thought process may be the cause for a patient's inability to comprehend written material and follow through with the exercise. Also, a debilitating depression may make it difficult for someone to have the motivation to stick with an exercise.

It is important to look around the room and be mindful of who may be struggling with the exercise. Provide individual help where appropriate. Don't just look for people who aren't working. Some people may be writing and, from a distance, may appear to be fine. When you look at what they are writing, you may find that it is psychotic or that they have no comprehension of the exercise. The point is, never assign an exercise and then leave the room or concentrate on something else, such as your own paperwork. Circle the room and take a good look at what patients are doing; make yourself available for questions and individual tutoring.

Oral Exercises

Oral exercises are those structured exercises that do not require writing. Some examples in this book include Stating Your Case, some parts of the Creating the Support Team series, and conflict resolution skits, What's in a Hospital? and What Is Relapse Prevention?

Again, with oral exercises, be mindful of anyone who may have a limited command of the English language. You will need to employ all your group-work skills to handle overactive and underactive patients, impulsive patients, and grossly psychotic patients.

Role-Play

Role-play is standard fare in didactic groups. Some examples of exercises in this book in which role-play is key include parts of Creating the Support Team, and conflict resolution skits Old Maid with a Twist and Rewriting Your Life.

Props can be useful in role-play. For example, play telephones are useful when role-playing the invitational call for Creating the Support Team. I will often begin by doing the role-play myself. I will start with someone who is more proficient at it and later include less proficient people. Sometimes I ask one or two proficient patients to sit next to someone who is lower functioning so that they can feed them lines when they get stuck.

For example, I once ran an assertiveness training group in which one of the patients was having great difficulty refusing entry to her alcoholic friends who often came knocking at her door late at night. She was chronically suicidal and identified this stressor as one of the causes for her suicidality. The group room in which we were working was adjacent to a kitchen with a door. I asked three strong-willed men in the group to play the part of her friends. They got cups of water to simulate alcoholic beverages. The patient was sent into the kitchen with the remaining three patients, who were to coach her in ways to keep these men from entering the kitchen when they knocked to come in. Not only did the patient improve her ability to assert herself, but the other three patients learned from the experience as well (as observed by their comments at the end of the group when I asked what they learned). Additionally, one of the men developed an awareness of the impact of his actions on others (he, at times, imposed his will on others). Last but not least, a good time was had by all—including me.

Therapeutic Games

Therapeutic games, as well as movie clips, help to make a full day of therapy—day in and day out—bearable. No one could stand four hours' worth of intense psychotherapy, even if they were highly motivated, psychologically sophisticated, and possessed the ability for delayed gratification, which is not the case for many people in a day hospital. Therapeutic games provide fun along with difficult therapeutic work. Another advantage to therapeutic games is that dynamics often are played out without the conscious awareness of the patients. They do not have to confess their dynamic shortcomings during the game, they only have to act them out. The discussion comes afterward (therapeutic games should always end with process). Some examples of therapeutic games included in this book are Self-Expression Game, The Balancing Act, Crisis Game, and the various games in Games Made Therapeutic.

I also include a discussion of ways to adapt for your use existing therapeutic games not necessarily constructed for a psychiatric population. Some therapeutic games, however, such as those that involve jumping from trees into other peoples' waiting arms, are simply unsuitable for this population (and do not meet the insurance requirements of the hospitals, in all probability!).

In my experience, several key things are required to make therapeutic games work. First, designing them and setting them up require a lot of work. Second, it is important to screen out people who cannot handle the therapeutic game and run an alternative group for them. Possibilities include people who cannot handle the game for physical reasons (such as someone who experiences dizziness for an eyes-closed exercise) or people who can't handle the demands of the game for psychological reasons (too psychotic or developmentally disabled to comprehend). There is nothing worse than running a game with a handful of people who can play full out and another handful of people who have no idea what's going on!

Third, be mindful of space when designing therapeutic games. Make sure you choose indoor games that can be used in the winter, summer, or in inclement weather. If the game requires people to be out in the hallways, make sure that they will not be too noisy or disruptive if there are other practitioners in adjoining offices conducting therapy sessions. Also, be aware of patients who tend to wander if the game requires them to leave the room. It is much harder to supervise people once everyone leaves the group room.

Use of Metaphor

By "use of metaphor" I am referring to the use of some special prop or set of props to metaphorically illustrate a point. Examples in this book include Shades of Gray . . . and More: Exploding Dichotomous Thinking, Singing in the Rain: From Adversity to Advantage, Murphy's Law Revisited, and Captain of the Ship.

In Shades of Gray . . . and More, the metaphor of color is used to help contrast "black-and-white thinking" (dichotomous thinking) with creative thinking (involving many colors). In Singing in the Rain, high-heeled shoes, a pencil, and a tuning fork are props used to illustrate that there is more than one way to see things. Murphy's Law Revisited uses "Murphy's Law" as a springboard for discovering the "Murphy's Laws" that we invent for our own lives—those laws of doom that become self-fulfilling prophecies.

The lovely thing about metaphor is that it creates an image to help us remember the lesson. A personal example will illustrate this point. I used to attend an Episcopal church in which the rector gave phenomenal sermons. He had a gift for using metaphors to illustrate his points. Once he used the metaphor of a child who attended a banquet with all kinds of exotic foods who was discontented because there was no boxed macaroni and cheese. I remember the lesson that he taught because that image sticks in my mind.

Using metaphors and props also makes the groups more fun, a central ingredient to holding people's attention (especially if their attention span is short).

THERAPEUTIC THEMES

This book is divided according to therapeutic themes. Each section begins with an introduction of that theme; hence, I will not elaborate on the themes right now. The themes are broad-scoped in order to include the largest number of patients possible. Most people have problems with self-esteem. Everyone needs to learn how to prevent a relapse. Everyone needs to set goals. By using therapeutic themes that fit the needs of most of the people in the room, you will have an easier time justifying each patient's inclusion in that group in your progress notes. Some insurance companies now require that a note be written for each patient, which lists the treatment plan goal and objective that was addressed by the group. Since each person's treatment plan is different, this can be very challenging. Groups addressing broad themes make that job a little easier.

You might decide on totally different therapeutic themes, which is fine. Adapt and invent.

HOMEWORK

Homework is employed in some of the groups, particularly the movie groups. I created homework in order to extend the therapeutic work outside of the day hospital. I also wanted to give people time—days—to think about some of the issues.

I always explain that homework in the day hospital is not like homework in school. You can't fail, you don't get punished if you don't do it, and you don't get a grade. Patients are also encouraged to help one another. Asking for help is not cheating. I emphasize these points frequently in order to allay anxiety about homework.

Homework is rarely collected and always discussed. People are welcome to join in the discussion whether or not they did the homework. On occasion, I find out in the beginning of the group that virtually no one did the homework. In that case, I give the group ten to fifteen minutes to do the homework before beginning the discussion.

The homework rarely involves more than the writing of two or three paragraphs about something. For some people, this will be monumental. Others who feel the need to do more automatically extend the assignment to suit their needs.

Chapter 2

Theory and Technique: The Context for Creative Groups

It is beyond the scope of this manual to offer a thorough discussion of any one theory or set of techniques. Reference will be made throughout to books that address these more thoroughly. The notes at the end of this chapter as well as the bibliography at the end of this book help expand the reader's knowledge of particular theories discussed.

Before one can make use of the outlines provided in this manual, they must be put in the context of theory and technique. First, it is important to understand some of the basic tenets of conducting group therapy. There are a number of books written on this topic, including Kathy Kaplan's *Directive Group Therapy*[1] and the various books written by Irvin Yalom, perhaps the most famous theortician in the area of group psychotherapy.[2] For those readers who are new to group therapy, Kaplan's book is a wonderful primer, not only because it provides useful information but because it is provided in a way that helps the beginner feel supported. Being a beginner can be fraught with anxiety. The beginner often wonders, "Am I doing it right?" "Will everyone be able to tell that I'm not sure what I'm doing?" "What if something unexpected happens in the group?" Kaplan's book coaches the beginner through these hurdles.

Irvin Yalom's *The Theory and Practice of Group Psychotherapy* is a very well-known book in which the author describes his basic model of interpersonal group psychotherapy. He utilizes the "group-as-a-whole" model. In this model, interventions are based not only on the psychodynamics of each of the individual participants but on the effect that those psychodynamics have on the group. The group itself is facilitated in such a way as to make *it* the healer, rather than the therapist. For example, a person who exploits others, thereby incurring the anger of other group members, might be encouraged to ask others how they feel about him and to receive feedback about his behavior with the group members. It is a *here-and-now* model; that is, one that focuses on the present rather than the past. Yalom also presents his famous discussion of ten curative factors in groups (imparting information, instillation of hope, universality, altruism, the corrective recapitulation of the primary family group, development of socializing techniques, imitative behavior, interpersonal learning, group cohesiveness, and catharsis). Yalom explains in detail how each of these factors helps to effect a shift in character structure (the nature of one's personality) and how, consequently, group therapy aids in improving the quality of life for group members. Yalom's book may be the most famous and the one most often referred to by other group theorists; hence, it is highly recommended to the beginning group psychotherapist.[3]

Of course, reading is only the tip of the iceberg. The real learning occurs in practice. You have to actually run groups to truly learn how to be a group therapist. One might begin by observing groups, either behind a one-way mirror or by sitting in the group itself. When ready, one might then move on to be a cotherapist in a group with an experienced therapist. Cotherapy can be tricky as it involves a cooperative arrangement between two therapists without the luxury of constant discussion about how to work together. It is like dancing. The two dancers must have a sense of how to move together without having a discussion about it while on the dance floor. However, they can certainly discuss it off the dance floor and practice again, knowing that in time, they will be able to feel each other's moves and have an intuitive sense of how to dance together. By being cotherapist with different therapists, one gets a chance to experience how different people work. One is also likely to experience the full range of difficulties in such an arrangement, which is what makes one an experienced therapist.

In addition to understanding the basic vicissitudes of running a group, one also needs to practice from a *theoretical orientation*. This may include psychoanalytic, psychodynamic, cognitive-behavioral, existential, interpersonal, and others. The beginner should read about various theories to discover which one feels right and which one he or she is most interested in pursuing. It is important to have a solid theoretical framework from which one works when running groups or doing any type of therapy.

Here a comment is in order about what works best in day hospital groups. Mental health practitioners today must take economic realities into account when determining their interventions. In this day of managed care, brief therapies are called for to maximize the use of the insurance company's dollar. In many cases, authorization from the insurance company is required before a client can be seen and the practitioner can be assured of payment. This means that interventions of which the insurance companies disapprove mean less business and less income. Brief therapy techniques, such as those discussed in Budman and Gurman's *Theory and Practice of Brief Therapy,*[4] are designed to maximize the possibility of concrete and measurable changes in behavior over a relatively short span of time. Some examples of brief therapy models include cognitive-behavioral and behavioral techniques,[5] here-and-now models of family therapy such as structural family therapy,[6] and biological interventions such as psychotropic medication and electroconvulsive therapy (ECT).[7]

Additionally, lengths of stay in both inpatient units and day hospitals are relatively short. When I began my work at the Adult Acute Day Hospital of the University of Medicine and Dentistry in New Jersey, the average length of stay was four weeks. A mere three years later it was cut in half to two weeks. Even over a four-week period, one can't expect much patient progress utilizing a model of intervention that usually takes years, such as analysis. With only two weeks, and sometimes less, one must work as efficiently as possible. This is reflected in the various discussions about techniques utilized in inpatient groups. Much of what applies to inpatient groups can be applied to day hospitals, as both use short lengths of stay for people who are acutely distressed. Where appropriate, I include phenomena discussed in writings about inpatient groups in my discussion of day hospital groups.

Brabender and Fallon discuss nine models of intervention in their book titled *Models of Inpatient Group Psychotherapy.*[8] These models are structured interventions that focus largely on what brought the person to the hospital. They help the patient manage problem behaviors; that is, those behaviors that brought them into the hospital. The focus is on here-and-now matters. The idea behind a group is to have members learn from one another. Brabender and Fallon discuss the *interpersonal model* of group therapy, which is based on the Sullivanian notion that all psychological problems are social problems insofar as they disrupt our ability to relate to others.[9]

Irvin Yalom's *group-as-a-whole* model is an interpersonal model. In his book, *Inpatient Group Psychotherapy,* Yalom discusses some of the differences between outpatient and inpatient groups. Much of what he says can be applied to day hospital groups as well. One difference is the short-term time frame.

> Inpatient group therapists cannot work within a longitudinal time frame; instead, they must consider the life of the group to last *a single session.* This necessity suggests that they must attempt to do as much effective work as possible for as many patients as possible during each group session. The single-session time frame dictates that inpatient group therapists strive for efficiency. They have no time to build the group, no time to let things develop, no time for gradual working through. Whatever they are going to do, they must do it in one session, and they must do it quickly.
>
> These considerations demand a high level of activity. . . . Inpatient group therapists must structure and activate the group; they must call on members; they must actively support members; they must interact personally with patients. . . .
>
> *Nor is there a place in inpatient group psychotherapy for the non-directive leader!*[10] [italics mine]

Why? In addition to time constraints, there is the degree of pathology of the patients. Patients need external structure, which, according to Yalom, facilitates internal structure. Yalom also distinguishes between two types of groups: one for higher-functioning patients and one for lower-functioning patients. Indeed, the needs of the person who is grossly psychotic and is working on reality testing are far different from the needs of an articulate individual whose struggle is with suicidal ideation. Yalom encourages the members of higher-functioning groups to set their own agendas. There is less external, staff-imposed structure for the higher level group because they have the internal structure from which they can set their own agendas and pursue their own goals. The lower-functioning group, however, needs more structure from the staff. For example, you might use a *round robin technique* (one in which you go around the room and ask everyone to speak to a specific issue) rather than letting people choose if and when they will speak. Or, you might facilitate a *sentence completion,* such as "Today I'm feeling _____."[11] Of course, there are times when everyone on the unit or in the day hospital meets together, as in, for example, community meetings.

Kathy Kaplan's *Directive Group Therapy* focuses on running groups for lower-functioning patients, something which is not emphasized in this book. She defines "lower functioning" in terms of the Axis V diagnosis which describes the GAF (General Assessment of Functioning). GAF is scored from 1 to 100 with 1 being the lowest functioning and 100 being the highest (in reality, no one ever gets a 1 or a 100). She recommends that the techniques described in her book be directed toward patients with a GAF between 11 and 30. These people usually exhibit psychosis or other severe impairment. Goals might include attending to a task, speaking once in the group, improving reality testing, or improving basic ADLs. She describes a number of group activities that can be used for this population such as bean bag toss, working on plants, etc.[12] One of the convenient things about working with this population is that the same kinds of groups can be run repeatedly without boring the patients (within reason). Someone who is struggling to attend to a task or to stop listening to internal stimuli is not likely to complain that "We just did the gardening group last week"; indeed, they may not even remember that you did the group last week. Higher-functioning patients, however, will complain if you run the same group this week that you ran last week. This creates a different challenge and a demand for a wider variety of groups. It is my hope that the outlines for groups in the latter half of this manual will help to some degree to alleviate that problem.

Yalom also stresses the importance of meeting in a room with closed doors and discouraging late arrival. Open spaces that allow people to come and go at will during the group create a lot of disruption that jeopardizes the flow of the group.[13]

What sometimes makes this difficult is that doctors and other staff, whose schedules are tight, often feel the necessity to pull people out of group in order to get all of their work done in a timely fashion. The trick here is to negotiate with them for the maximum possibility of fulfilling the principle of least disruption. Perhaps it would be possible to negotiate about which groups a patient will be asked to miss. Perhaps the patient may be seen in a waiting room before the group starts rather than being pulled out of the group. A group facilitator may need to be a master negotiator on a constant basis with regard to this matter.

The following scenario is a disaster. Perhaps it is a day when attendance is low to begin with, maybe because the census is low or because the weather is bad. Whatever the reason, one starts the group with five people and, within fifteen minutes, various professionals (doctor, nurse, dietician, etc.) come in, interrupt the discussion, and ask certain patients to leave. By the time the group is half done, only two people may be left after several interruptions. The facilitator may feel like declaring an end to the group and turning on the TV. The patients would also be annoyed. This can't be allowed to happen.

When designing the physical space of the day hospital, group privacy also must be taken into account. In our facility, the group room was placed in the middle of the day hospital surrounded by peoples' offices. It was as if the group room was the center of a wheel. There was no way to get to the offices other than to walk through the group room. The door would open and close repeatedly. Heads would turn as people passed through. Patients with short attention spans would be lost, and all patients complained that no one respected their space. The situation was hard to correct in our facility because of the physical setup. Hopefully, the physical setup of the program in which you work (or will work) will be different. If not, have frequent staff discussions about this problem. Ask people to move in and out of their offices during the breaks between groups, to close the door very quietly, and so forth. Don't wait until you are completely exasperated to baddress the matter. Bring it up right away, and bring it up often.

Alonso and Swiller discuss the benefits of groups in the day hospital and the various approaches to groups that seem to work best.

These are brief therapy approaches such as behavioral approach, medication groups, family support groups, and activity groups. The behavioral groups include those that address the specification of goals, assertiveness training, desensitization for people with phobias, anxiety management training, as well as educational groups and groups to improve ADLs (activities of daily living) such as grocery shopping, use of transportation, money management, etc. Medication groups focus on patient discussion of the effects and side effects of their medication as well as the importance of medication compliance. Multiple family groups focus on providing education and support to families of the patients, while activity groups are task oriented with the goals of increasing concentration and improving communication skills. Notice that these are brief therapies. They are short term, behavioral, and aim for concrete and specific results.[14]

THEORETICAL ORIENTATIONS

Now that we have discussed some general issues related to group therapy in the day hospital setting, let us move on to discuss specific theoretical orientations in group work and how the outlines in the latter part of the manual might be used in the context of these orientations.

The Psychodynamic Models

The psychodynamic models include a wide variety of theories, among them Freudian, object relations, self-psychology, and developmental. Proponents of these theories include Sigmund and Anna Freud, Karen Horney, Erik Erikson, Harry Stack Sullivan, Margaret Mahler, Otto Kernberg, Heinz Kohut, and others. A full discussion of these theorists is well beyond the scope of this book. The reader may refer to the bibliography for further reading.[15-20]

I will briefly mention two models as examples. The *object relations model* was developed by various theorists, including Mahler and Kernberg. This model was developed in an attempt to have a more interpersonal method of analysis, as it was felt that *drive theory,* which emphasized the internal drives (ego, id, superego, sexual drives, and aggressive drives), was lacking in its understanding of the interpersonal problems confronting patients. Object relations theory discusses the manner in which the psyche develops as a relational phenomenon. It discusses the move from early infancy, in which the child is said to live in its own world and be oblivious to the sense that there is anything out there that is "not me," to the splitting off of the self from the mother. Key notions discussed include *splitting, projection,* and *projective identification.* Splitting and projection refer to the idea that we disown parts of ourselves and project those parts onto others. Often, we split off parts of ourselves that we find dangerous. For example, the infant may experience rage when not attended to immediately, which happens some of the time to all infants. It is too threatening for the infant to feel enraged with the mother, who it sees as the vehicle for survival; hence the rage is split off and projected outward. Over the course of its development, the child should be able to reincorporate the rage as a part of himself again. Likewise, the infant may split off the "good mother" from the "bad mother" in order to continue to experience pleasure through the mother at a time when it may not have the psychological defenses to tolerate pain and frustration. Again, in a healthy individual, the "good" and "bad" mother will eventually be integrated as the child is able to tolerate frustration and anger without psychological disintegration. If development goes awry, this integration may not occur. This often leads to the development of borderline pathology.

Projective identification is another key phenomenon in object relations theory. It is a defense in which an intolerable feeling or intolerable notion about the self (let's say murderous impulses) are projected onto another person. Then, through various subtle means, the patient manages to provoke the object (person) on which he has projected this feeling to behave in exact accord with the forbidden phenomenon. For example, someone who cannot tolerate their seductive side might provoke someone else to be seductive, projecting their seductiveness onto them. Typically, they will attempt to "destroy" that part of themselves by criticizing and otherwise trying to "get rid of" that which was projected onto the other person. In this case, the patient might be highly critical of someone else's seductiveness.

Brabender and Fallon offer a nice discussion of object relations theory that makes it easy for the beginner to understand, as some of the original writings may be difficult to plow through, in all honesty.[22] They discuss object relations theory in the context of general systems theory, which emphasizes the impact that internal dynamics have on the group and vice versa. Group interventions consist largely of clarifying interpretations, that is, interpretations that help group members understand what they are acting out in the group process.

Erikson's *developmental model*[23] is another psychodynamic theory. Erikson's model outlined the psychological tasks children progress through at specified ages as they grow into mature adults. Most of us fail to pass through the first four stages completely without some problems. The problems we encounter with these stages determine where we are *developmentally arrested.* Where we are developmentally arrested will determine the shape and characteristics of our personality as well as the nature of the interpersonal problems with which we will suffer. The first four stages include development of trust, resolution of conflict with authority figures (differentiation), development of identity, and development of competence. In an inpatient or day hospital setting, the arrest is often either in Stage One or Two (for borderlines, most often Stage Two). These conflicts are again acted out in the group and, through the use of clarifying interpretations, the group members are aided in resolving these conflicts.

Several problems are encountered in utilizing these types of approaches today. First, they tend to take a long time and, as we noted earlier, insurance companies prefer short-term therapy. If, as Yalom put it, we need to consider the length of the group to be one session, we must seriously consider what can be accomplished with these models in one session. Second, one way to determine the efficacy of a method is to review research that clearly demonstrates a concrete change in behavior or clear resolution of the presenting problem as a result of the intervention. Many of the terms utilized in psychodynamic theories are hard to define or operationalize. *Operationalizing* a term means that one defines it in a way that it is measurable and therefore amenable to empirical research. Terms like "projective identification" are not quantifiable. This does not mean that the interventions are not effective, just that they do not easily lend themselves to empirical research.

Having made these observations, I still would like to discuss the manner in which psychodynamic interventions might be used with some of the groups later described in this manual.

As noted earlier, projection is a defense used when an impulse, feeling, or idea becomes intolerable to the psyche. Working with the projection can be a psychologically safe means of helping the patient to work through "dangerous" concerns. In analysis, one way this is done is by the working through of *transference* (what Sullivan termed *parataxic distortion*). Projection is a form of transference in that the patient transfers personal thoughts and feelings onto the analyst and believes that those thoughts/feelings/characteristics actually reside with the analyst rather than with himself. The analyst utilizes the transference to help the patient eventually own those feelings for himself and thereby become a more whole person.

Movie groups offer the patients opportunity to project difficult thoughts and feelings onto a safe figure—a movie character. This is even safer than transferring the feelings onto another person, as a movie character is not going to object to the transference, while another person might say, "I don't do that! You're the one who does that!" Remember that in the day hospital, we tend to work with people who are regressed more significantly than neurotics who never require hospitalization. We tend to see people who are psychotic or suffering with significant personality disorders. They require stronger defenses to keep themselves from psychological disintegration. Projection is a lovely defense, and strengthening it by offering the patient a movie figure onto whom a difficult aspect of themselves may be projected is useful.

An example occurred with the group titled What's Wrong with This Picture? (page 143). The movie cut involved a character named Josh, the protagonist in the movie *Big,* starring Tom Hanks. In this sequence, Josh arrived at a party inappropriately dressed. People sniggered as he walked into the room. He then proceeded to exhibit other lapses in social graces, including licking the cheese out of the stuffed celery, dipping his vegetables five or six times in the dip after biting, flinging an unwanted corn cob to the side, and spitting out caviar while making a lot of noise about it. I asked the day hospital group the question, "What problems with social graces did you note here?" (this was a low-functioning group). To my surprise, they completely ignored the question and proceeded to discuss how unfair it was, in their eyes, that people laughed at Josh just because he was different. It became clear to me that Josh was, for them, the social outcast that they often feel they are themselves. He didn't "fit in" and they imagined that he really felt his lack of belonging. (This was clearly projection on their part, as it is obvious in the movie that Josh is completely unaware that he doesn't fit in.) We moved from a discussion of social graces to a discussion of how it feels to deal with the subtle signs of ostracism patients often experience when they are in public. They were barely able to touch on their own social awkwardness and the shame that they felt about this. By discussing Josh's social awkwardness and the reaction he induced in others at the party, they could begin to touch on this phenomenon in themselves.

Another example of the usefulness of projection occurred while running the group titled, Relationship and Risk (page 150). One of the movies utilized is *Ordinary People* and in one of the movie sequences the protagonist is nervous about seeing his psychiatrist for the first time. He then has a fairly disastrous first interview in which, among other things, the psychiatrist asks him questions that he is tired of answering and that he feels the psychiatrist should already know by having read his chart. Patients are offered the opportunity to comment on this sequence. It may be difficult for patients to criticize staff because they rely on staff for emotional succor, good care, etc. For some patients with personality disorders, who may have managed to anger family members and lose friends, the staff may be all they have in the way of caring relationships. This would make it hard to be critical. However, staff regularly do things that irritate patients, such as asking the same mental status questions repeatedly ("Are you going to make me count backwards by seven and spell 'world' backwards again?") or asking questions they should know the answers to if they took a look at the chart beforehand. By giving the patients an opportunity to comment on the movie psychiatrist's incompetence, they do not necessarily have to say directly that they do not like our incompetence. Yet they know that we are listening when they tell us about the movie characters.

Existential Model

The existential model of psychotherapy originated with existential philosophers including Kierkegaard, Nietzsche, and Heidegger as well as others. Analysts became concerned with the use and misuse of technique.[24] The question of *being* became an issue in psychotherapy when some analysts began to feel that therapy was becoming somewhat impersonal, or missing the boat in its attempt to understand the whole person. Rollo May put it very nicely in his book, *The Discovery of Being:*

> Can we be sure, one such question goes, that we are seeing the patient as he really is, knowing him in his own reality; or are we seeing merely a projection of our own theories *about* him? Every psychotherapist, to be sure, has his knowledge of patterns and mechanisms of behavior and has at his fingertips the system of concepts developed by his particular school. . . . But the crucial question is always the bridge between the system and the patient—how can we be certain that our system, admirable and beautifully wrought as it may be in principle, has anything whatever to do with this specific Mr. Jones, a living, immediate reality sitting opposite us in the consulting room?[25]

Concerns such as this led to an existential form of psychotherapy. Leaders in this field include Binswanger, Allport, Boss, May, and Yalom.[26]

One of the key constructs in existential therapy is that of *responsibility.* The nature of the human being is seen such that, with consciousness comes choice, and with choice comes the responsibility to exercise fully one's capacity to make choices. Pathology is seen as the limiting of one's ability to make quality choices by one's neurotic concerns.

Goldberg and Goldberg discuss distinctions between the analytic model and the existential model with its emphasis on intentionality and responsibility. They state that:

> The therapist's function is not to change the patient's behavior but to help him discover his intentionality so that he has more conscious choice about his behavior. Freedom and choice have

a psychogenic origin in that an appropriate mode of behavior is feasible only to the extent that it is conceptualized as a possibility; otherwise, it does not exist as a behavioral alternative.[27]

It is my personal sense that this is where analysts were always headed; it is the very point of analysis. However, the existentialists have, here, said so frankly and placed more emphasis on it.

Goldberg and Goldberg discuss various types of irresponsibility. One type of irresponsible behavior they describe is the assignment of causes for problems to external sources. This is typical, for example, of those with personality disorders. They will spend the therapy session complaining about others and insisting that their happiness lies with change in the others' behavior rather than their own behavior or point of view. If the therapist suggests that they might have something to do with the problem, the suggestion is often rejected.[28] People who do not accept responsibility for their own behavior are said to lack insight and it may be tough to work with them.

Goldberg and Goldberg describe two other kinds of irresponsibility: using one's inner life to avoid contact with the external world, and blaming one's self rather than taking responsibility for altering a situation.[29] Blame renders a kind of paralysis to the situation, whether one is blaming others or one's self. Blame is the opposite of owning responsibility for one's own dilemma. While the hallmark of blame is the inability to do anything about the situation, the hallmark of responsibility is "the ability to respond," to do something to change the situation. I can believe that I am unhappy because my boss is horrible (blaming others), because I am horrible (self-blame), or because I perceive the world in a manner that leaves me unhappy. In the latter case, I can change my perception, whereas there is nothing I can do about "being a horrible person." I might also change my behavior if it is provoking others to treat me in a way that leaves me unhappy. The last interpretation ("my perception/behavior makes me unhappy") gives me an avenue for change.

In a group setting, one will help patients to reclaim responsibility for their own behavior, hence freeing them from the ways they have paralyzed themselves with irresponsible perceptions. I once ran an open ended (unstructured) group in a day hospital. A patient I will call Mary paced around the room nervously as she complained bitterly about her weekend ordeal. Her aunt threw her out of the house and called the police following an incident in which she grabbed a large knife, began shaking nervously, and locked herself in the bathroom. She complained that her aunt was insensitive for throwing her out of the house and leaving her homeless. She spoke of her aunt's lack of understanding of her mental illness.

Therapist: Mary, let's stop for a minute to take another look at this. You're obviously upset about being homeless, and about the incident in general. That's very understandable. I'd like to help you make sure that nothing like this happens again. Usually, when there's a conflict, everyone plays some part in the conflict. It may seem more obvious what part some people play than others, but in my experience, everyone plays some part. Everyone brings something to the party, so to speak. What do you think you brought to the party?

Mary: Well, the knife, I guess.

Therapist: Uh-huh. And what effect do you think that had?

Mary: I don't know. (silence)

Therapist: Put yourself in your aunt's shoes. How would you feel if you came home and saw someone locked in the bathroom with a knife? What would you think?

Mary: I guess I'd think they were crazy.

Therapist: Yeah, it does fit the stereotype that people sometimes have, doesn't it?

Mary: Yeah. I guess I scared her.

From here the group discussion moved on to things patients do that inadvertently support the stereotypes people have about them. It was a productive discussion, whereas a discussion about how unfair it is that people stereotype them might have been less productive.

Goldberg and Goldberg state that the focus of attention in the group is at times on an individual, at times on a subgroup, and at times on the entire group. These shift from one to another, as in the above example, where the focus of attention was initially on an individual but later was on the entire group.[30]

Goldberg and Goldberg make some other distinctions between traditional analytic or psychodynamic group work and existential group work. They feel that the therapist tends to be more self-revealing and to more often express his/her own feelings in existential group work. They state that not all emotional reactions are historical, that is, based in transference. Some have "immediacy" and "presence." Emotional involvement of the therapist is essential to helping patients with these. They speak of responsible self-revelation, of course. For example, they do not advocate revealing one's own dynamic concerns where they have no therapeutic value to the group. As with all interventions, self-revelation must be done consciously and for sound therapeutic reasons. Goldberg and Goldberg also examine distortions and projections only insofar as they impede present relationships, not for curiosity about the past.[31] This, of course, is consistent with our earlier discussion of what is needed in a short-term therapy, which is focus on the here-and-now. The groups in Chapter 11, "Motivation," were designed in the context of an existential point of view.

Blame and irresponsibility are very tempting ways to deal with mental illness. It's easy to blame the illness and, in so doing, sentence the patient to a life of no possibility. This is not to say that one should encourage patients to do what is obviously beyond their reach. However, one should not encourage patients to do less than they can because they are "ill." When I conducted groups at the day hospital, I found that the patients were most responsive to the groups in the motivational series. I believe that they found it refreshing that someone encouraged them to stretch just a little beyond what they thought they could accomplish.

In the group titled, Beyond Survival: Creating a Life Worth Living (page 174), patients who hide behind their illness, rather than courageously stepping out, are confronted and challenged. The content of the movie as well as the questions reflect a bid for responsibility. The Captain of the Ship (page 190) is all about the concept of responsibility. The other groups give the patients the message that they can move forward in their lives, and they are responsible to do so.

As reflected in the quote earlier in this section, the goal of the work is to help the patients realize their "intentionality"; to "conceptualize appropriate responses as a behavioral alternative." The therapist's responses, therefore, should always be in line with that goal. For example, a patient once told me in group that she was not "normal." She was an intelligent, articulate, high-functioning woman with a bipolar illness. When I asked her to define normal, she stated that it meant being married, having a job, and having a house. I then asked her if she considered me normal, to which she responded, "Oh, yeah!" I told her that two out of three of those things were not true about me; at the time, I was not married and did not own a house. This opened up for her the possibility that she could be normal. Not only is this an example of opening up possibility for someone, but it is also an example of sharing one's self in a way that is therapeutic.

Cognitive-Behavioral Therapy (CBT)

Cognitive-Behavioral Therapy, or CBT, is a form of therapy that fits nicely into managed care guidelines. Why? It is short term. It aims for concrete and measurable results, which allows one to prove the efficacy of one's treatment. And it is a here-and-now method of therapy. Types of CBT include rational-emotive therapy, systematic rational restructuring, cognitive therapy, self-instructional training, and stress reduction training. Two important characteristics of CBT are that it is highly directive and homework is used a great deal. The goal of CBT is not to "cure" the patient but to increase his or her level of functioning through the methods of disconfirming cognitive distortions, creating new cognitions that are more empowering, and increasing insight by helping the patient understand the process by which cognitive shifts are made.[32]

I highly recommend reading the chapter titled, Refuting Irrational Ideas, in *The Relaxation and Stress Reduction Workbook* by Davis, Eschelman, and McKay.[33] I often recommend that chapter to my patients, as it is an easy-to-read, compact way of understanding the basic concepts of CBT. The homework page gives one a good feel for how homework is used in CBT.

When using CBT in groups, the focus is still on the individual. The group leader moves from person to person, helping them work through their homework or shift from a disempowering cognition to one more empowering. For example, if a patient states, "I just know I'm going to end up in the hospital again," the therapist might write that statement on the board and help the patient to see that this is a cognition that is running his or her life, one that becomes a self-fulfilling prophecy in many cases. The patient might be helped to make a cognitive shift: "With good support, I don't have to be in the hospital again." The patient will be encouraged to note the difference in the feelings generated by more empowering cognitions.

Beck discusses *depressogenic thinking:* cognitive distortions that are common for those suffering from depression. For example, *catastrophizing* is a process by which the depressed person tends to see everything as a catastrophe waiting to happen. *Dichotomous thinking* is a kind of "black and white," "either/or" kind of thinking that ignores the gray areas in life. People are either all good or all bad, work is perfect or no good, etc. These two types of thinking work together, in that, often, if one condition is not met, a catastrophe will occur. For example, "If I can't take lithium, I'll be in the hospital." The patient here must be helped to conceptualize other possibilities: "If I can't take lithium maybe I can take another drug like Depakote or Tegretol"; "Maybe the doctor can adjust my lithium"; "Maybe I can still be helped on an outpatient basis."

The group in this book titled Shades of Gray . . . and More: Exploding Dichotomous Thinking (page 103), addresses this *depressogenic error* (cognitive error commonly experienced by those who are depressed). The Blue Car Syndrome (page 106) addresses overgeneralization, an error in which one or two experiences are used to make gross generalizations that limit one's possibilities. For example, having relationship problems with one or two people "proves" that, "Nobody likes me," or "I'm no good." Singing in the Rain: From Adversity to Advantage (page 107) addresses fatalistic thinking, a cognitive error in which one takes a fatalistic approach to things ("I just know we're going to get into an accident"). Murphy's Law Revisited (page 111) addresses catastrophizing.

As mentioned, with CBT the therapist works one-on-one, even in the group setting. Why bother with the group? First, it is efficient to teach a lot of people at once, and efficiency is important in the current economic climate. Also, people learn from one another. Everyone hears as you help one patient correct a cognitive distortion; hence, everyone learns. Further, group members can help each other. When someone is unable to generate a more empowering cognition (and this happens often), other group members can help with ideas. This teaches patients that they can consult with one another in their everyday lives when they are unsure how to generate solutions to their problems.

In addition to one-on-one correction of cognitive distortions and follow-up with homework, one can encourage new behavior to be tried outside of the day hospital setting (or inside the inpatient setting). Suggest the goal of sitting in the cafeteria with a person the patient does not know well and holding a conversation in order to refute the idea that "No one likes me," then follow up the next day to see how the new behavior worked. If it didn't turn out well, the patient is in danger of using it to strengthen disempowering cognitions ("See, I knew no one would like me"). This needs to be corrected quickly.

I would like to mention that movies may be used here, if desired. One can select movie cuts in which characters exhibit cognitive distortions and then ask the patients to correct these distortions. Stories can be used in a similar way. There is a suggested reading from C.S. Lewis's *Chronicles of Narnia* in the group titled, Singing in the Rain: From Adversity to Advantage.

Related techniques include the focal problem approach or psychosocial therapy and behavioral therapy. Behavioral therapy is a broad term that includes the use of token economy, systematic desensitization to address phobias, multi-modal therapy, and others. The common features of the behavioral therapies, as in CBT, are that they are empirical and action oriented, focus on behavior, evaluate antecedents and consequences of behavior, and have an ahistoric focus (here-and-now). The psychosocial approach is a problem-solving approach that focuses on daily activities or skills needed for daily living. In the focal problem group that utilizes a problem-solving approach, the group members identify a problem in as much detail as possible, discuss the ways that the problem has been dealt with in the past, explore potential solutions to the problem, settle on actual solutions, and later evaluate the workability of those solutions once they are tried.[34] In a short-term setting such as a day hospital, aftercare may be arranged to further address the problem. One of the main methods used to help the person define a problem and its solution is *partializing,* that is, breaking a problem down to smaller parts that can be more easily managed.

The relapse prevention groups and goal-setting and support groups in this book focus on problem solving. For example, The Mountain Exercise is about defining a goal, partializing it, and defining a strategy for addressing each part (page 97). The Crisis Game (page 85) is a fun way to anticipate problems and develop solutions before the problems, or crises, occur. People are often hospitalized when they are overwhelmed with a crisis. Helping people to anticipate solutions in advance may prevent future hospitalizations. Ideally, the underlying message patients always hear in such groups is: "Problems can be solved. It is not necessary to go into the hospital, decompensate, or act out in destructive ways in response to problems."

When discussing the psychodynamic approaches to therapy, I discussed some of their disadvantages in a short-term setting. To avoid the implication that behavioral approaches are a panacea for psychological problems, I offer this quote from Goldberg and Goldberg:

> The focal problem approach is particularly relevant to people who suffer chronic unmitigated frustration and psychological impotence—to people who have not experienced themselves constructively affecting their environment and do not have confidence in being able to do so in the future. . . . However, I do not contend that a cognitive approach to life problems is a substitute for personal insight or intensive psychotherapeutic experience.[35]

In other words, one must consider the limits of what can be accomplished with these approaches. Problem solving and/or elimination of symptoms that result in hospitalization will relieve some suffering and, perhaps, buy someone the luxury of further work of a deeper nature in the future—work that might facilitate a shift in character structure. Not everyone will be interested in doing that work, nor should it be attempted in a short-term setting. It is important, however, to be aware of the limits of short-term methods and the possibility of further work in the future to promote a better quality of life.

APPLYING THEORIES TO GROUP WORK: AN EXAMPLE

I have briefly described the therapeutic models that influenced the creation of the groups in this book. I would now like to demonstrate how they might be applied to the group work itself by taking a small section of one group and discussing the interventions from the standpoint of psychodynamic therapy, CBT, and existential therapy. We will use the group titled Driving Miss Daisy: Accepting Support (page 166).

Let us imagine that you are running this group. You have just shown the first movie clip in which Miss Daisy refuses to meet Hoke, the chauffeur her son just hired for her. You ask the group the first question: "What do you think of Miss Daisy's attitude? How do you think she feels?"

Psychodynamic Model

Note that the question invites projection. The group is invited to project their own feelings onto the character of Miss Daisy.

Patient 1: I think she feels angry.

Therapist: Why?

Patient 1: Because her son is running her life. No one has the right to do that. She didn't ask for the driver.

(Here you might hypothesize that this patient is angry about others, perhaps parents, making decisions for him. Perhaps his parents are overresponsible. Or perhaps he is acutely aware that others his age make their own decisions and, like Miss Daisy, he feels ashamed.)

Therapist: How about others? What do others of you think?

Patient 2: I agree. She's mad.

Patient 3: She doesn't want to meet the driver.

Therapist: What do you think of that?

Patient 3: Well, she doesn't have to be nasty. He's only trying to help her.

Patient 1: But she never asked for him!

Therapist: So, for some of you, Miss Daisy's son arouses some strong feelings of anger. Some of you feel that Miss Daisy should be allowed to make her own decisions, while others of you feel that Hoke is there to help. Let's talk about these two feelings.

(One might hypothesize that group members are expressing ambivalent feelings about dependency: they feel secure with it but also feel threatened due to the loss of autonomy.)

One thing to note: You can continue as directed in the book or you can veer off in your own direction. Perhaps you might ask: "How do *you* feel about Hoke?" or "How do *you* feel about Miss Daisy's son?" The idea is not to be enslaved by the outline. Rather, you should use it as a guide and as a way to "kick start" a discussion about whatever is germane to the patients' well-being.

Cognitive-Behavioral Therapy (CBT)

Let us return to the first question you asked the group after showing the movie clip: "What do you think of Miss Daisy's attitude? How do you think she feels?"

Patient 1: I think she's angry.

Therapist: Why?

Patient 1: Because her son is running her life. No one has the right to do that. She didn't ask for a driver.

Therapist: Yes, that's very good. You noticed that Miss Daisy didn't ask for a driver. You also said, "Her son is running her life." Let's look at that in terms of the CBT model we've been using. (Goes to board and writes:)

EVENT   *THOUGHT*   *FEELING*

So, Patient 1, what was the event?

Patient 1: Miss Daisy wouldn't meet the driver.

Therapist: Right. Because . . .

Patient 1: 'Cause she didn't want one.

Therapist: OK. Great. So the *event* that made Miss Daisy mad was that . . .

Patient 1: Her son hired a driver.

Therapist: Right! (Writes this under *EVENT.*) And what *thoughts* do you think Miss Daisy had about that? Anyone?

Patient 2: He has no right to run my life.

Therapist: OK, let's put that down. Other ideas?

Patient 3: My son thinks I'm dumb.

Therapist: OK. (Writes it down.) (Takes down other thoughts.) And these *thoughts* leave Miss Daisy feeling how?

Patient 1: Mad.

Patient 2: Sad.

Patient 4: Suicidal. (Laughter from others.)

Therapist: Well, if Miss Daisy felt bad enough, she could feel suicidal. So let's put that down. Now. The key is to change these thoughts to more empowering ones so Miss Daisy won't feel so bad. This doesn't mean that Miss Daisy has to agree to the driver, just that she might not feel so hurt by the whole situation, or feel the need to be rude. So let's look at the *thoughts* we outlined (reads them). What might be some more empowering thoughts that would lead Miss Daisy to feel better?

Patient 2: Well, she might think that her son means well. He's just trying to help.

Therapist: OK. So let's do this again.

EVENT	THOUGHTS	FEELING
Miss Daisy's son hires a driver	"He's just trying to help."	

What other thoughts?

Patient 2: Maybe the driver won't be so bad.

Therapist: OK. (Therapist takes down more new thoughts.)

Therapist: And how might someone feel after having these thoughts?

Patient 1: I still think she'd be mad. But maybe less mad.

Therapist: OK. Less mad. What else? Would she feel suicidal, Patient 4?

Note that projection is still used in CBT. For example, in the movie, one doesn't get the sense that Miss Daisy is suicidal. However, Patient 4 may be struggling with suicidal feelings. These were projected onto Miss Daisy. The therapist validated the projection (hence validating the patient). The difference between this and the last scenario is that the CBT method was used instead of an open discussion to resolve the struggle.

Again, remember to be flexible with these outlines, one could spend the entire group session on this one clip. One might move on to thoughts the patients have about their own dependency utilizing the CBT method. It is not necessary to ever even get to movie clip two!

Interpersonal Model (Group-as-a-Whole)

Here we will need to use a different scenario in order to create a brief but clear illustration. The key here is to focus more on the interaction between the patients.

Therapist: What do you think of Miss Daisy's attitude? How do you think she feels?

Patient 1: I think she's angry.

Therapist: Why?

Patient 1: Because she doesn't like her son running her life. She never asked for a driver. (Talks awhile, monopolizing the group.)

Therapist: I wonder what others think? (Silence, then . . .)

Patient 1: She feels sad, too. (Continues talking.)

Therapist: Great, Patient 1. Anyone else have any ideas? . . . Patient 1, I notice you've been doing all the work for the group.

Patient 1: Well, no one else is talking.

Therapist: What does that feel like, when you have to carry the group like that?

Patient 1: I don't like it. C'mon guys.

Patient 2: I figured he was doing just fine so I didn't need to say anything.

Patient 3: Yeah, me too.

Patient 4: I can't think of something good to say, like Patient 1. It takes me a long time to think of something to say. I'm afraid everyone will think it's stupid.

Therapist: So, Patient 1, you feel a little frustrated sometimes when you do all the talking. And the others of you feel hesitant about talking, especially when you notice that Patient 1 is doing a good job. Let's keep talking about this. I think it's interesting that our theme for today is support. Sometimes it feels good to let others, like Patient 1, support us. Sometimes it doesn't feel good. And then there's the matter of how those who are supporting us feel. Let's hear more about this. Patient 4, you said that it's hard for you to think of something to say; that it takes time for you to do that, and that you're afraid what you say might be thought of as stupid. Can you tell us more about that?

(The therapist is being directive due to the short-term nature of the day hospital and in order to challenge the patient who is not likely to be spontaneous. Whether or not this line of intervention would continue depends on the patient's response.)

I used this scenario because it is a frequent one encountered in the day hospital: one or two patients do a lot of the talking while the others, perhaps patients struggling with the negative symptoms of schizophrenia, do almost no talking. Patients often at once invite the overresponsibility of others and yet resent it. You see how the group process was interwoven with the theme. In the group-as-a-whole model, you can keep asking patients to give feedback to one another, making them the healers of one another.

Existential

Therapist: What do you think of Miss Daisy's attitude? How do you think she feels?

Patient 1: I think she's angry.

Therapist: Why?

Patient 1: Because her son is running her life. No one has the right to do that. She didn't ask for a driver.

Therapist: So you feel that Miss Daisy's son is running her life.

Patient 1: Yes.

Patient 2: He has no right to control her.

Therapist: Are you saying that Miss Daisy is not in control of her life?

Patient 1: Well, yeah. The car was taken away from her. That's not right.

Therapist: What do others of you think?

Patient 2: I agree. (Others agree.)

Therapist: Well, suppose Miss Daisy really can't drive now. Maybe she really doesn't possess the ability to do it, even though she wants to. Does that mean she's lost all control of her life? Is her life over?

(Patients are quiet, as it's a tough question. Therapist lets them think.)

Patient 3: No. She's still alive.

Therapist: Um. What *can* she control?

Patient 2: She could pick the driver.

Patient 3: True. (More silence.)

Therapist: Are there other things she can control? Is driving the only thing in her life?

Patient 1: I guess not. She runs the house, bosses people around.

Therapist: Yeah. So I guess she controls something, huh? I guess what I'm asking is, even if you have some kind of problem, like losing an arm or having a disease or losing your coordination, can you still make something of your life?

The therapist used the movie clip and responses to open up an existential discussion about how the patients can create meaning in their lives and how they can be responsible for their lives in spite of their problems.

ABOUT MOVIE GROUPS

"Movie groups" use cuts from movies as springboards for discussion. They are quite useful because they make a group more interesting. Additionally, a clip from a movie can often convey an emotion or concept far more powerfully than mere words. While it takes time to invent a movie group, once it is created it can easily be used repeatedly.

Preparing the Group

The first step in inventing a movie group is to decide on the theme for the group. Some examples include intimacy, family relations, self-esteem, and overcoming obstacles to one's goals. The movie should be the medium through which your therapeutic goal is expressed. If you think of a theme for which you cannot think of a movie, consult employees of video stores who tend to be familiar with a variety of movies. Ask others you know. This will be particularly helpful if you don't frequent the movies yourself.

Once you select your theme and the movie you will use, view the movie in its entirety if you have never seen it before. Then go over the movie a second time, stopping at scenes that you feel relate to your theme. Write down the counter numbers denoting where the cuts begin and end. For each cut, generate a broad question (or more than one question) for discussion. For example, suppose my overall theme is "handling adversity." I decide to use the cut from *Cinderella* in which her stepsisters tear her dress apart, preventing her from going to the ball. In despair she runs out into the yard, falls on her knees, and says that she has nothing to believe in anymore. I might ask the questions: "When have you been in despair? How did you behave at that time?"

After you have formed the question, arrange the cuts and questions so that there is a natural progression from one cut to the next. That may not always mean that the cuts are presented in the order in which they occur in the movie. Remember it's the theme that prevails (the therapeutic content), not the movie!

The last two things to do are to prepare a homework question, if you wish, and to prepare a snappy title for the group.

Running the Group

The following outline can be used for running the group:

   I. Introduction of theme
  II. Introduction of movie
 III. Movie cuts and questions
 IV. Homework

Introduction of Theme

After mentioning the theme, I often find it useful to obtain opening feedback from the group about the theme. For example: "Today we are going to examine the issue of courage. What do you think courage is?" Leave plenty of time for this discussion, even if it means that you will not get to all the movie clips. I have run many groups in which I did not show all the clips I had planned to show. The groups were still successful. I will expand upon this later.

Frequently the opening question will be a request to define something, as in the example above. Patients often begin by attempting dictionary-type definitions. This is fine. I quickly move, however, to asking for a description of what the term means to them ("I'm not looking so much for a dictionary definition as I'm looking for what courage means to you. What does it mean to you personally? Where has it played a role in your life?").

You will realize when this part of the group is complete. Perhaps most everyone will have spoken. Perhaps there will be a longer silence. Or someone might say something that proves to be a perfect segue to the first cut.

Introduction of Movie

No matter how popular the movie or story, never assume that everyone knows the story. This is especially true for people who spent years being psychotic or who come from chaotic family backgrounds where no one read stories to them. I use Walt Disney's *Cinderella* for one group. I have yet to run this group and find that everyone is familiar with the story of *Cinderella.* Of course, there is the issue of potential embarrassment or shame because of this. For that reason, if it is a very popular story, I refrain from asking, "Who is not familiar with this movie?" I simply ask someone to summarize the story.

I often ask two or three people to summarize the story. After the first person speaks, I ask if anyone would like to add something to this person's description because, usually, the summary is rather sparse. If the two or three summaries are somewhat disjointed and do not convey the basic theme of the movie itself, I finish with my own summary.

Movie Cuts and Questions

Be sure to introduce each cut by giving some background. For example: "In this cut Cinderella speaks with her stepmother and stepsisters about going to the ball." Remember that the cuts will feel different to you than they do to someone who has never seen the movie. You automatically place them in context with the rest of the movie. Others do not know the characters' names or how they got to be where they are. Think about the details that need to be shared. For example, suppose you use a movie in which there is a divorce early in the action. In your first cut, you show a scene in the marriage. Your second cut shows the protagonist flirting with someone else. Your viewers may wonder if there was a divorce, separation, or if this is an extramarital affair. Your introduction would then be: "Sandra was divorced and lived alone for six months. In this next cut she meets Tom and is attracted to him."

You can also pose questions before showing the cut. For example: "As you watch this scene, look for evidence of codependency in the relationship." Also, do not be afraid to rewind the film and play a cut again if you think this will be helpful. If, for example, in the above situation no one picks up any codependent behavior, run the clip again.

Patients often project their own issues onto the film. This makes it possible for them to discuss some issues they might otherwise feel too threatened to approach. One of the consequences of this phenomenon is that the patient may extract a theme that you never saw or planned to discuss; in other words, they may see something entirely different from what you see. If it is way off base, deal with it quickly and move on (for example, if it is paranoid or psychotic in nature). If others relate to it and pick up on the discussion, be willing to change the theme. The patients ultimately will use the movie in the way that serves them best. This is where we need to "listen with the third ear."

For patients whose thinking is more concrete, you will receive superficial and concrete answers. If you ask, "What did you see in that?", they will reiterate the facts of the scene ("She got on the bus and went to her mother's house"). Do not be discouraged by this even if it occurs frequently. Support the person and his or her view and continue to ask for feedback from the group until you get a more abstract answer.

If you find that the discussion has been good and you are running out of time, you can simply follow your outline as long as it goes, *or,* better yet, decide which cuts to eliminate. You might skip a couple of cuts and show your last cut, for example. It is an on-the-spot decision that you'll have a feel for when the time comes.

Remember to consider technical matters. Make sure that the volume is loud enough for everyone to hear, including older people with hearing problems. When fast-forwarding, you can choose to turn the TV off (no picture) or leave it on (fast-moving picture). If the distance between the two scenes is short, I would choose the latter; however, I would not fast-forward until the discussion is complete for two reasons. First, patients will pay attention to the pictures on the screen rather than to what their fellow patients are saying. Second, your own attention is diverted. You are trying to find the right "next spot" while listening to someone. You would be better off just listening. If the next clip is far from the previous one, I would turn the TV off. This is less distracting. You can also fast-forward during the discussion and switch your attention to the TV when you get close to the cut. I make these recommendations with the assumption that your budget does not allow you to pay someone to copy all of the cuts onto a tape so that you can simply have everything on one tape with one cut following another. If you have money in the budget for this, go for it!

Homework

Be sure to leave plenty of time at the end for people to write down the homework question. You may think this only takes a minute. In reality, however, people will be slow to find their notebooks and pens, those who do not have paper and pen will need to obtain some from their peers, and people will write slowly. The process could take ten minutes or more.

Make sure you use the movie group no later than Wednesday if you plan a homework question to be reviewed on Friday. And do not forget to turn the lights back on when you write the question on the board!

EXERCISES

Now it is your turn to be creative and therapeutic. Choose one of the following exercises.

1. Take any movie clip mentioned in this book, or any other movie clip you are aware of that would be appropriate to use in a day hospital. Show it to the class. Create two questions that

you might ask after showing the clip. Explain why you would ask those questions. For what kinds of problems might this clip be useful?

Discuss typical projections that patients might make onto the character(s). Discuss why you think these projections are likely to occur.

2. Choose any exercise in this book and write a one-page hypothetical-process recording, in which you use CBT as your intervention.

3. Choose any exercise in this book and write a one-page hypothetical-process recording, in which you use the interpersonal model. Use one of the following scenarios:

   a. All of the group members are very quiet. No one seems engaged.
   b. One person is monopolizing the group, and everyone else appears to be annoyed.
   c. The group starts discussing something way off the topic.
   d. Someone is very hostile toward you and almost loses control. Everyone else is tense.

4. Discuss an existential problem that day hospital patients are likely to face. Create a part of a group using movie clips, stories, newspaper clips, games, etc.—whatever you like—to facilitate a discussion among the patients addressing this existential issue. Discuss your group with the class, explaining the rationale for what you created.

5. Form a group of four to six people. As earlier in this chapter, take one movie clip and question, then create three scenarios based on three different theoretical orientations/techniques. Feel free to include a theory not discussed in this book if you wish.

NOTES

1. Kaplan, Kathy L., *Directive group therapy.* Thorofare, NJ: Slack Inc., 1988.

2. Yalom, Irvin D., *Inpatient group psychotherapy.* New York: Basic Books, 1983; Yalom, Irvin D., *The theory and practice of group psychotherapy.* New York: Basic Books, 1983.

3. Yalom, Irvin D., *The theory and practice of group psychotherapy*, pp. 3-83.

4. Budman, Simon H., and Gurman, Alan S., *Theory and practice of brief therapy.* New York: The Guilford Press, 1988.

5. See Beck, Aaron T., *Anxiety disorders and phobias: A cognitive perspective.* New York: Basic Books, 1985; and Beck, Aaron T., *Cognitive therapy of depression.* New York: The Guilford Press, 1979. Aaron Beck is among the most well-known of the cognitive behavioral theorists, especially for his scales, such as the Beck Depression Scale, which offer a way to measure progress in therapy. This, of course, is very appealing to those in managed care environments, as it gives them a measurable way to prove that they are making a difference.

6. See Minuchin, Salvador, *Families and family therapy.* Cambridge, MA: Harvard University Press, 1974. Minuchin has written other books, but this is probably his most famous and the one people frequently use to learn about structural family therapy.

7. See the brief article on day hospitals in Harold Kaplan and Benjamin Saddock's *Comprehensive group psychotherapy.* Baltimore, MD: Williams and Wilkins, 1993.

8. Brabender, Virginia, and Fallon, April, *Models of inpatient group psychotherapy.* Washington, DC: American Psychological Association, 1993.

9. Brabender and Fallon, *Models*, pp. 55-111.

10. Yalom, *Inpatient group psychotherapy*, pp. 106-108.

11. Yalom, *Inpatient group psychotherapy*, Chapters 5 and 6.

12. Kaplan, *Directive group therapy*, Chapter 3.

13. Yalom, *Inpatient group psychotherapy*, pp. 109-110.

14. Alonso, Anne and Swiller, Hillel, eds., *Group therapy in clinical practice.* Washington, DC: American Psychiatric Press, Inc., 1993.

15. Freud, Sigmund, *Abstracts of the standard edition of the complete psychological works.* New York: International University Press, 1973.

16. Horney, Karen, *Collected works of Karen Horney.* New York: W.W. Norton, 1985.

17. Erikson, Erik H., *Identity and the life cycle.* New York: W.W. Norton, 1980. Also, Erikson, Erik H., *Childhood and society.* New York: W.W. Norton, 1985. The latter is a collection of essays that help to illuminate his theory.

18. Sullivan, Harry S., *The interpersonal theory of psychiatry.* New York: W.W. Norton, 1953; Sullivan, Harry S., *Collected works.* New York: W.W. Norton, 1965, c. 1940-64.

19. Mahler, Margaret S., *The psychological birth of the human infant: Symbiosis and individuation.* New York: Basic Books, 1975. Mahler is famous for the subject of this book. Also, Mahler, Margaret S., *The selected papers of Margaret S. Mahler, MD.* New York: Jason Aronson, 1979.

20. Kernberg, Otto, *Borderline conditions and pathological narcissism.* Northvale, NJ: Jason Aronson, 1985. Kernberg, until recently, was probably the biggest name in work with borderlines. Now that the shift of emphasis is being made from psychoanalytic models to behavioral models, Marsha Linehan has become the big name in working with borderlines. She is known for her invention of dialectical

behavioral therapy. Also, for familiarity with Kernberg's work, see Kerberg, Otto, *Object relations theory and clinical psychoanalysis.* Northvale, NJ: Jason Aronson, 1986, c. 1984.

21. This discussion is taken from a synopsis of these models offered by Brabender and Fallon, *Models*, pp. 115-241.

22. Ibid.

23. Brabender and Fallon, *Models*, pp. 243-319.

24. May, Rollo, *The discovery of being: Writings in existential psychology.* First edition. New York: W.W. Norton, 1983.

25. May, Rollo, *The discovery of being*, p. 38.

26. My personal recommendations for readings in this area are the aforementioned book by Rollo May, which gives a nice overview of both the existential philosophers and the existential psychotherapists, explaining how the former influenced the latter; and Yalom's *Existential psychotherapy* (New York: Basic Books, 1980). I found Yalom's book to be very readable and quite moving. For fun, you might wish to read Yalom's novel, *When Nietzsche Wept* New York: Basic Books, 1992. This is a gripping novel that beautifully portrays the attitude of the existential psychotherapist.

27. Goldberg, Carl and Goldberg, Merle Cantor, *The human circle: An existential approach to the new group therapies.* Chicago: Nelson Hall Co., 1973, p. 41.

28. Goldberg and Goldberg, *The human circle*, p. 42.

29. Goldberg and Goldberg, *The human circle*, pp. 43-44.

30. Goldberg and Goldberg, *The human circle*, pp. 90-91.

31. Goldberg and Goldberg, *The human circle*, pp. 139-144.

32. Brabender and Fallon, *Models*, pp. 499-605

33. Davis, Martha, Eshelman, Elizabeth Robbins, and McKay, Matthew, *The relaxation and stress reduction workbook.* Oakland, CA: New Harbinger Publications, Inc., 1988. I also make frequent use of Copeland, Mary Ellen, *The depression workbook.* Oakland, CA: New Harbinger Press, Inc., 1992. This is a workbook that gives concrete suggestions for relapse prevention for anyone suffering from depression or bipolar illness. A videotape by Copeland offers the same material (available through New Harbinger Publications, Inc.). Another book I like to use for people with anxiety disorders is Edmund J. Bourne, *The anxiety and phobia workbook* (Oakland, CA: New Harbinger Publications, Inc, 1990), which won the coveted Franklin Award and is one of the best books I've ever seen on this subject for patients. For a more clinical discussion of CBT, refer to the aforementioned books by Aaron Beck.

34. Brabender and Fallon, *Models*, pp. 157-161 and 419-498.

35. Goldberg and Goldberg, *The human circle*, p. 151.

Chapter 3

Beginning the Day

Most day hospital programs have rituals to begin the day. These may include serving a continental breakfast, having a brief meeting to review the schedule for the day, going over special events, introducing new people, and so forth. Below is a list of other ideas for opening the day:

1. Have everyone report on something in the news. Have newspapers available for that purpose.
2. Have a piece of trivia or a new word for the day.
3. Mention something that occurred in history. When I was in eighth grade, I had a history teacher who began each class by telling us something that happened in history on that particular date. You may not be able to be as specific (unless you can find a book that includes a calendar listing historical events), but it would be easy to report one item of history each morning.
4. Have people do some light stretching (nothing that requires them to get on the floor or to be too flexible). Some head and neck stretches, shoulder stretches, and a bend or two at the waist would suffice.
5. Ask the question, "What are you looking forward to today?"
6. Have everyone set a small goal for the day.
7. Have a brief discussion about one relapse prevention technique, such as limiting or eliminating alcohol consumption.
8. Have a culinary tip for the day.
9. Have a brief discussion about a motivational quote, such as "We have nothing to fear but fear itself."

Do not engage in activities that are likely to lead to heavy processing if you are having a short opening meeting. For example, do not have patients discuss the previous evening's activities lest it turn into an unintended group therapy session. Keep the topics concrete and/or light. Clarifying the agenda for the day, rules, and other aspects of structure, combined with starting off on a light note sets a good tone for the rest of the day.

Chapter 4

Relapse Prevention

Relapse prevention is an excellent therapeutic theme to use in your program for several reasons. Clinically, it makes sense to empower people to prevent future relapses. Financially, managed care companies are going to appreciate interventions designed to keep someone out of the hospital in the future. Relapse prevention is a topic that is germane to everyone in the day hospital; there is no one for whom this category of groups would not be justified.

Relapse prevention is a very broad therapeutic theme which may include information about medication, information about lifestyle changes that reduce the possibility of relapse, groups about handling crises that may increase stress and promote relapse, etc.

The first group, What Is Relapse Prevention?, is a brainstorming exercise. What I like about this is that patients sometimes have idiosyncratic ways of preventing personal relapses that clinicians would rarely consider (e.g., getting a pet). By letting the patients create the list, their own creative strategies are brought out in the group in addition to the traditional strategies. Also, allowing patients to brainstorm gives them ownership of the strategies. Last but not least, they have to stay awake in order to *say* the strategies, whereas they can fall asleep while *listening* to us.

The next group, Creating the Support Team, covers at least three sessions (I have often used four to five sessions for this series). I have tried several ways of handling the paperwork over a period of weeks (I ran my relapse prevention groups once a week). I used to hand out one worksheet at a time. This usually meant that people lost them one at a time. Next I tried giving patients the entire package. I did this partly because, in a short-term day hospital program, people come and go quickly, which meant people often left before I finished the entire series. I wanted them to have the materials for the entire series so that they could use them post-discharge. The problem with this method was that people would forget to bring the packets in with them, no matter how many times I told them not to forget. My next and last strategy was to hand out entire packets and to collect them at the end of each group. So far this has worked pretty well. It also allows me to look over their work one more time and write personal comments, which the patients have traditionally found very useful. I include further tips about this series in the group instructions themselves.

The Hospitalization Review is very useful for people who are not actively psychotic and have a reasonable degree of insight. In my experience, most people learn at least one new thing about how to prevent future relapses or recognize relapses early on after participating in this group. One word of warning: some people become agitated during this exercise because they find it too painful to think about the times when they were psychotic or suicidal. Also, please keep in mind my comments in the introduction about being aware of people with reading problems as well as people who are not proficient in the English language. For your convenience, both the Hospitalization Review and parts of Creating the Support Team are translated into Spanish. The parts of the latter group that are translated are those parts that the patient will use.

What's in a Hospital? is another brainstorming exercise. This exercise is excellent for surreptitiously getting patients to discuss the secondary gains involved in hospitalization. Occasionally, the list of "good" things about being in the hospital has been twice as long as the list of "bad" things. This evidence for secondary gain provides a great springboard for discussion about secondary gain. (I have had many other times in which the "bad" things list is longer. This creates opportunity to discuss motivation for staying out of the hospital.)

The Crisis Game was designed for lower-functioning patients whose judgment may be poor. I found, however, that everyone had fun with the game. Since the questions were designed for lower-functioning patients, consider running separate games for higher-functioning and lower-functioning patients. If possible, it is a good idea to use crisis situations that resemble those crises that led to the patients' hospitalizations and/or crises that they face in their current lives.

The Crisis Skit is a good activity for higher-functioning patients; it requires too much ingenuity to be useful for lower-functioning patients. The nice thing about the Crisis Skit is that it allows patients to project whatever personal concerns they have onto the skit. You can turn it into a psychodrama group if you wish, having patients take turns playing out various solutions to the problem.

There are many other things that you can do for relapse prevention. For example, you might create an entire series in which you discuss a different aspect of relapse prevention each week. You might design a special group for people who have just completed their first hospitalization. The possibilities are endless.

WHAT IS RELAPSE PREVENTION?

Preparation

None!

Activity

Begin by asking patients to define "relapse prevention." They will probably attempt dictionary-like definitions. That is OK in the beginning. Help them to move toward more personal definitions after that.

Ask the patients to brainstorm about behaviors that prevent relapse. Have someone write these on the board. Be sure the list includes:

1. Taking medications as prescribed. Explain to the patients why taking medications when you feel bad and discontinuing when you feel good does not work.
2. Decreasing isolation. Patients might say such things as, "see friends, go places, don't stay alone," etc.
3. Keeping a positive outlook on life.
4. Having emergency numbers available.
5. Seeing a therapist.
6. Getting an appropriate amount of sleep.
7. Eating well.
8. Exercising.
9. Cultivating interests unrelated to mental illness (e.g., a hobby, religious activity, sports, etc.).
10. Having others available for support. Creating a support team (see pages 51-66) is a great tool for relapse prevention.

After creating a list, allow the rest of the time for the group to elaborate on any part or parts of the list.

CREATING THE SUPPORT TEAM

(3 sessions or more)

Preparation

You will need copies of the worksheets that follow. You may also like to use play telephones for the role-play that occurs over the phone. The toy phones that have ringers and play tunes such as *London Bridge* add an element of fun to the group. They are not expensive.

Opening Discussion

Begin by discussing the concept of a support team. A support team is a handful of people known to the patient who will provide ongoing support for him or her and will step in to provide extra support during a period of crisis. There are some important characteristics to know about a support team.

1. The support team comprises people known to the patient. These are people the patient trusts. They should be known to be reliable.
2. The support team is not responsible for the patient's well-being. The patient is responsible for that. The support team is just that—support. This point is very important not only to reinforce the patient's ultimate responsibility for him or herself but also to reassure the support team member that the patient is not putting his or her life in the support member's hands.
3. The patient will define his or her needs for the team. Each team member will choose which, if any, of those needs s/he wishes to provide.
4. People are free to "resign" from the support team. If the people enlisted are reliable, they will "resign" responsibly (e.g., not in the middle of a suicidal crisis).
5. The ideal support team consists of three to six people.

Patients should understand that support teams are created while they are doing well. The idea is to be prepared for a time in the future when there may be a crisis.

Activity 1

The patients will need to educate the members of their support teams about their symptoms. In order to do this, the patients first will have to be aware of their own symptoms.

Instruct the patients to fill out Worksheet #1 (SYMPTOMS I EXPERIENCE WHEN I AM NOT WELL). Be sure they use lay-person's terms (e.g., "I am preoccupied with my own thoughts and stare into space constantly" rather than "I am internally preoccupied"). They should also describe symptoms that are concrete and measurable, which will be observable to the members of the support team.

The sheets should be completed in pencil. Drastic revision is usually needed. People have a hard time with "concrete and measurable." Sometimes they have a hard time even identifying any of their symptoms, especially if they were in denial about the need for hospitalization. ("I went into the hospital because they believed my wife.")

The bottom part of the sheet has blanks for emergency numbers. Patients can complete this section at home if they do not know some numbers, such as parents' or spouse's work numbers. Everyone should be made aware of the hospital emergency number.

Activity 2

Patients should next fill out Worksheet #2 (IDEAS FOR WAYS TO SUPPORT ME). Patients need to be aware of the kind of support they desire prior to asking for that support. They also need to communicate their desires in a way that is understood by others. The worksheet will help with these matters.

The right side of the sheet indicates the desired support person for each item. That person may or may not agree to do it, but the patient can ask for that specific person.

Activity 3

Review the outline to the invitational call with the patients. Take plenty of time with this and encourage questions.

Do a lot of role-play using the play telephones. This will take a long time, maybe even more than one session. Patients often struggle enormously with this even when following the outline. They may need to rehearse repeatedly.

It is very important not to rush this part. If patients start making calls from home prematurely, the calls will go badly. This often results in losing what small support network they had to begin with as the only two or three people who might be on their support team turn them down. Don't ask them to try to call from home until you are convinced they can do this successfully.

You may need to spend time on the second part of the worksheet as well. It is typical for patients' support networks to be extremely small. People who are depressed often lose what friends they have because their friends can't tolerate their depression and because patients don't keep up the contact. Schizophrenics are often shunned by others and sometimes live in their own psychotic world. Recovering addicts have to give up their entire network of addicts. They must start over without the aid of their drug of choice to help them feel comfortable with meeting others. Because of these situations, patients will probably tell you that they cannot do the worksheet because there is no one to support them. This often calls for the remedial step of looking at how to expand one's support network. It may mean that it takes awhile before the first invitational call can be made at home. You want to be careful about this, however, as some patients have a support network they haven't acknowledged. Those people simply need help to acknowledge who is supporting them already.

Activity 4

The next step is to practice for a group meeting. Once all of the individual members of the team are on board, a group meeting is held to educate the group about symptoms and enlist their support. Use Worksheets #4 and #5 (AGENDA FOR GROUP MEETING and PUTTING IT ALL TOGETHER: SAMPLE GROUP MEETING) for this purpose.

Begin by reviewing Worksheet #4. Encourage questions and discussion. Then move on to Worksheet #5. If possible, do not choose people with flat affect, poor concentration, or inability to read for this first example. The example does not come across well under those circumstances. You want people to get a *feel* for the group meeting.

Entertain questions and discussion. Then form another group that will ad lib their own meeting. Choose someone to play the patient who you think will be able to do this independently in the relatively near future. Provide plenty of coaching and feedback for the patients during this exercise.

Homework

Finally, patients should be able to do the various parts of this exercise in real life, specifically the invitational calls and the group meeting. Do *NOT* assign these for homework for the entire group at once. Follow people individually and assign to them what they are ready to handle. Monitor progress closely.

When assigning the invitational calls, begin by having the patients make one call. They should come back and report on that call before making another. This gives you a chance to catch the call if it is a disaster before they repeat the experience.

Worksheet #1

SYMPTOMS I EXPERIENCE WHEN I AM NOT WELL

1.

2.

3.

4.

5.

6.

7.

8.

IMPORTANT NUMBERS

Hospital Emergency Number: _____

Therapist's Number: _____

_____

_____

_____

Worksheet #1

SAMPLE: SYMPTOMS I EXPERIENCE WHEN I AM NOT WELL

1. I eat very little—only one small meal per day.

2. I don't shower or brush my teeth.

3. I stay in my room for most of the day.

4. I say very little.

5. I cry a lot.

6. Sometimes I have thoughts about killing myself. (Ask me—I'll tell you.)

7.

8.

IMPORTANT NUMBERS

Hospital Emergency Number: <u>123-456-7890</u>

Therapist's Number: <u>Mary Jones   234-5678</u>

<u>Dr. Smith   345-6789</u>

Worksheet #2

IDEAS FOR WAYS TO SUPPORT ME

WHAT   WHO

  1.

  2.

  3.

  4.

  5.

  6.

  7.

  8.

  9.

10.

11.

12.

Worksheet #2

SAMPLE: IDEAS FOR WAYS TO SUPPORT ME

WHAT	WHO
1. Come to my house and cook a meal with me.	Mom
2. Let me eat at your house.	Mom, Nancy
3. Be able to talk on phone for about fifteen minutes when I'm feeling down.	Marge, Tom, Hank
4. Call me to get me out of bed until I can do it myself.	Marge
5.	
6.	
7.	
8.	
9.	
10.	
11.	
12.	

Worksheet #3

INVITATIONAL CALL

1. Ask the person if this is a good time to talk. If not, schedule another time.
2. Tell the person that you are doing well. Discuss the ways that your life is going well if you are able to do so genuinely. This will help him or her to realize that you are not making an emergency call. It will also set an optimistic tone for the call.

   If you are not doing well this is not the time for the invitational call. Talk about why you are not well instead, and do the invitational call another time.
3. Explain that you are in the day hospital and that you are creating a support team. Explain that a support team is a group of people that provide ongoing support to you and that also provide extra support when you are not doing well. Emphasize that you are completely responsible for your own well-being and that you simply are looking for some people to support you. Give the person a chance to ask questions and reassure him or her about the role if need be.
4. Invite the person to be on the team. Explain that s/he will have the choice to support you in whatever way is desired and that the ways can be spelled out specifically by you and by the team member.
5. If the person accepts, explain that there will be a group meeting of all support persons to explain everything. Find out when the best times are for the individual to have a meeting.

   If the person says no, thank him or her for his or her time. Do not be crushed. Some people are scared to be part of a support system. This is not your fault.
6. Always be sure to thank the person.

ADDITIONAL NOTES

PEOPLE I PLAN TO CALL

Name	Number	Result (Yes/No)

Worksheet #3

SAMPLE: INVITATIONAL CALL

Friend: Hello?

Patient: Hello. May I speak with Nancy?

Friend: This is Nancy.

Patient: Hi, Nancy. This is Loretta.

Friend: Hi, Loretta. How are you?

Patient: I'm doing really well.

Friend: Oh yeah?

Patient: Yeah. I was discharged from the inpatient unit five days ago and I'm in the day hospital now. I don't have thoughts about killing myself anymore and I'm not crying all the time. The medication's really working.

Friend: That's terrific.

Patient: Thanks. Nancy, do you have a few minutes for me to tell you about a project?

Friend: Sure. Go ahead.

Patient: Well, something they taught us to do at the day hospital is to create a support team.

Friend: A what?

Patient: Support team.

Friend: What's that?

Patient: Well, it's a small group of people who support you in little ways day to day and who are also available in a crisis. For example, support team members might be available for phone calls or go to the movies when you're down or something like that. Also, if you ever get sick again, support team members know what symptoms to look out for. They can call it to your attention early and

Patient: support you in getting help right away, before you end up back in the hospital. Of course, I'm responsible for my own well-being. The support team, however, can help me out.

Friend: I see.

Patient: The idea is to build your support team while you're well so you have help close at hand if you get sick.

Friend: Gotcha.

Patient: Well, Nancy, I'd really love it if you'd be one of my support team members. I think you'd be great. You support me already.

Friend: I'd love to, Loretta. What do I have to do?

Patient: Well, once I get five people to agree, I'm going to have us all meet together to discuss the details further. Are weekends good for you for a meeting?

Friend: This weekend I'm away. Next Saturday is OK.

Patient: Great. I'll let you know once I've spoken with the others.

Friend: OK.

Patient: Thanks a lot Nancy. I do appreciate it.

Friend: Sure, Loretta. I'll talk to you soon.

Patient: OK. Bye.

Friend: Bye-bye.

Worksheet #4

AGENDA FOR GROUP MEETING

1. Introduce people to one another if they don't know each other.
2. Thank them for being there.
3. Explain that you are creating a support team and what a support team is (a group of people that will provide ongoing support and will also provide extra support in times of trouble).
4. Explain that you want the group to be aware of your symptoms when you are not well so that they can help you. Hand out copies of Worksheet #1 (SYMPTOMS I EXPERIENCE WHEN I AM NOT WELL). Go over each of the items, making sure they understand what you wrote. Ask them if they notice any symptoms that you left off the sheet because sometimes others can see things that you may not be able to see yourself, especially when you are sick. If they mention other symptoms, have them added to the sheet (make sure you have pencils or pens handy for everyone).
5. Hand out copies of Worksheet #2 (IDEAS FOR WAYS TO SUPPORT ME). Go over the sheet and ask if people would be willing to provide those items of support to you. Make sure that you and they are specific about who is going to provide what. It is fine for more than one person to provide a specific item of support. Additionally, group members way wish to offer ways of supporting you that are not on your list. You may accept these, of course, if you wish. Be sure to allow people to refuse to do something if they do not want to do it. Try not to take it personally if they do—it is not a reflection on you.
6. Sum up the meeting and its results.
7. Thank everyone again for coming to the meeting. Remember that you can never say "thank you" too many times.
8. Have refreshments and have fun!

Worksheet #5

PUTTING IT ALL TOGETHER: SAMPLE GROUP MEETING

Patient: I think most of you know each other. Do you two know each other?

Mary: No, we haven't met. I'm Mary.

John: Hi, Mary. I'm John.

Mary: Nice to meet you.

John: Nice to meet you.

Patient: I really appreciate you guys coming out here and I especially appreciate your willingness to support me. This is what's going to help to keep me out of the hospital in the future.

Bill: No problem. We're glad to support you.

John: Yeah.

Patient: Well, even though I spoke with each of you about this on the phone, I'd just like to go over once more what a support team is about. I want to emphasize that I'm not making you all responsible for my life or my well-being. I'm in charge of that. But having your help, especially if I start to go downhill, might be enough to keep me out of the hospital. What we'll do today is we'll all agree on the various ways that each of you will support me. No one is forced to do anything they don't want to. The meeting will give me a clear idea of what I can depend on you for. It will also help you if we clarify the nature of your support so that this doesn't get overwhelming or out of hand for anyone.

I want to pass around a list of my symptoms. These are the things that happen to me when I'm starting to get psychotic. I think it's important for you to be aware of these symptoms because, when I start to get psychotic, I often can't see it. If you all start to see me doing these things on the list, like not eating, talking to myself, and spending days in my room, you know I'm in trouble.

Bill: What should we do when we see you like this?

Patient: Well, the first step would be to talk to me about it. If I can hear you, I'll call my doctor right away for help. If you find that I'm too far gone to be able to help myself, you could call the emergency number on the bottom of the sheet. They'll take over from that point on—you don't have to do the work of the professionals.

Incidentally, I signed release of information forms for all of you with my therapist and psychiatrist. This means that you are free to talk to them in a crisis if you need to, and they will be able to give you information.

John: So we don't have to try to counsel you or anything? Not that I don't want to help, but I wouldn't know what to do.

Patient: You're right, John! You're not supposed to be in that position. If you need professional help, call the professionals and they'll take over.

By the way, are there any symptoms or behaviors any of you see when I get sick that I left off the list?

Mary: Yeah. I was just thinking that your hygiene is usually bad when you get psychotic. You don't shave or shower. Sometimes you're scared to shower.

Patient: OK. Add that to your lists. Anything else?

(Silence)

OK. Let's move on to the list of ways you might support me. The things that would help me the most would be if I could have a ten- to fifteen-minute phone conversation with someone when I'm anxious or lonely and if someone would come over and cook and eat with me when I start to go downhill. I stopped eating the last two times I was hospitalized. I think that if someone was with me I'd eat.

Mary: I'm right next door. I'm usually home around dinner time. I'd be glad to come over whenever I can, to cook and eat with you. Or, if you want, you can come over and eat with our family.

Patient: Thanks, Mary.

Bill: I could talk with you on the phone sometimes. You know that I work long hours and I'm often not home, but whenever I am I'd be glad to talk with you if it will help.

Patient: Thanks.

John: Yeah, you can call me too. I don't mind.

Patient: Thanks.

Joe: I'm not sure I'd know what to say if you were getting crazy—no offense.

Patient: Don't worry, Joe. I'd just need some reassurance if I'm anxious. Or if I'm isolating myself you might suggest I go out to see someone or do something.

Joe: I don't know. I'm kind of nervous about it.

Patient: That's OK, Joe. You don't have to do this if you're not comfortable.

Joe: I'd give you a ride to the emergency room like last time if that would help.

Patient: Great. That ride was literally a lifesaver.

Joe: You're welcome.

Mary: Just let us know what you need and if we can help, we will.

Patient: Thanks a lot. So Mary, John, and Bill will be available for talking on the phone, Mary will be available for meals, and Joe will help out with a ride to the emergency room if I need it. Well, again, I really appreciate you guys. It means a lot to me.

I made a cake and there's some coffee. Who wants some?

Hoja de Trabajo #1

SINTOMAS QUE SIENTO CUANDO NO ESTOY BIEN

1.

2.

3.

4.

5.

6.

7.

8.

NUMEROS IMPORTANTES

Numero de Urgencia del Hospital: _____

Numero del Terapista: _____

_____

_____

_____

_____

Hoja de Trabajo #2

IDEAS PARA METADOS DE DARME APOYO

QUE   QUIEN

1.

2.

3.

4.

5.

6.

7.

8.

9.

10.

11.

12.

Hoja de Trabajo #3

LLAMADA DE INVITACION

1. Preguntale a la persona si este es un buen tiempo para hablar. Si no, programa otro tiempo.
2. Di le que te esta llendo bien. Hablen de las formas en que te esta llendo bien en tu vida si esto es algo que puedes hacer sinceramente. Esto le ayudara a realizar que tu no estas haciendo una llamada de urgencia. Esto tambien le establecera un tono optimistico a la llamada.

   Si no te esta llendo bien este no es el tiempo para hacer le llamada de invitacion. En vez, habla de las razones porque no estas bien y haz la llamada de invitacion en otra ocasion.
3. Explica le que tu estas en el "day hospital" y que estas formando un equipo de apoyo. Explica le que el equipo de apoyo es un grupo de personas que regularmente te proveer apoyo ye que dan apoyo adicional cuando no te esta llendo bien. Da enfasis que tu eres completamente responsable por tu propio bien-estar ye que estas buscando gente que simplemente te apoyen. Da le la oportunidad de hacer preguntas y asegura le de su papel si es necesario.
4. Invitale ala persona que sea porte de el equipo. Explica le que ellos podran escoger la forma que quieran de ofrecer apoyo y que estas formas seran especificamente delineadas por ti y por ellos.
5. Si la persona acepta, explica le que habra una reunion del grupo para que todas las personas de apoyo cubran a todo. Averigua los mejores tiempos para que ellos tengan una reunion.

   Si la persona dice que no, da le las gracias por su tiempo. No estes desilusionado. Algunas personas tienen miedo de ser parte de un sistema de apoyo. Eso no es tu culpa.
6. Siempre aseguara te de darle las gracias a la persona.

NOTAS ADICIONALES

PERSONAS QUE PLANEO LLAMAR

Nombre	Numero	Resultado (Si/No)
_____	_____	_____
_____	_____	_____
_____	_____	_____
_____	_____	_____
_____	_____	_____
_____	_____	_____
_____	_____	_____
_____	_____	_____
_____	_____	_____
_____	_____	_____
_____	_____	_____
_____	_____	_____
_____	_____	_____
_____	_____	_____
_____	_____	_____
_____	_____	_____
_____	_____	_____

Hoja de Trabajo #4

AGENDA PARA LA REUNION DEL GRUPO

1. Introduce a la gente si no se conocen.
2. Da les las gracias por estar presente.
3. Explica les que etas formando un equipo de apoyo y lo que es un equipo de apoyo (un grupo de gente que regularmente proveeran apoyo y que tambien daran apoyo adicional en tiempos de dificultad).
4. Explica qu tu quieres que el grupo este enterado de tus simtomas cuando no estas bien para que ellos te puedan ayudar. Reporte copias de las Hoja de Trabajo #1 (SINTOMAS QUE SIENTO CUANDO NO ESTOY BIEN). Cubre cada de talle, asegurando te que ellos entiendan lo que has escrito. Posiblemente queras elaborar en algunos de los detalles. Preguntales si ellos han notado cualquier otro sintoma que no escribistes en la hoja porque algunas veces otros puenden ver cosas que tu no puedes ver por ti mismo, especialmente cuando estas enfermo. Si ellos mencionan otras sintomas, haz que los agregen a la hoja (asegurate que tengas lapizes o lapizeros para todo el mundo).
5. Reporte copias de la Hoja de Trabajo #2 (IDEAS PARA METADOS DE DARME APOYO). Da le un repaso a la hoja y pregunta si la gente esta disponible a proveer esos metodos de apoyo para ti. Asegurate que tu yellos sepan especificamente quien va proveer que. Esta bien que mas de una persona provee un metodo de apoyo especifico. Adicionalmente, miembros del grupo quizas queran ofrecer metodos de apoyo que no estan en tu lista. Tu puedes aceptar estos, claro, si quieres. Aseguarate de permitir a la gente de nagarse a hacer algo si no lo quieren hacer. Trata de no tomarlo personalmente si hacen esto—esto no refleja en ti.
6. Resume la reunion y sus resultados.
7. Dale las gracias a todos por venir a la reunion. Acuerda te qu nunca se puede decir "gracias" denasiadas veces.
8. ¡Tomen refrescos y diviertanse!

Hoja de Trabajo #5

PONIENDO LO TODO JUNTO: EJEMPLO DE LA REUNION DEL GRUPO

Paciente: Creo que la mayoria de ustedes se conecen. ¿Ustedes dos se conocen?

Maria: No, no nos emos conocido. Yo soy Maria.

Juan: Hola, Maria. Yo soy Juan.

Maria: Gusto en conocerlo.

Juan: Gusto en conocerlo.

Paciente: Yo aprecio mucho que ustedes han venido y aprecio especialmente su buena voluntad de darme apoyo. Esto es lo que me va a ayudar mantenerme fuera del hospital en el futuro.

Guillo: No hay problema. Estamos contentos de darte apoyo.

Juan: Si.

Paciente: Bueno, aunque hable sobre esto por telefono con cada uno de ustedes, quisiera repasar otra vez lo que es un equipo de apoyo. Quiero dar enfasis a que no los estoy haciendo responsable por mi vida o mi bien-estar. Yo estoy encargado de esto. Pero teniendo su ayuda, especialmente si comienzo a decaer, puede ser suficiante para montenarme fuera de hospital. Lo que vamos hacer hoy es ponernos de acuerdo en los diferentes metodos de que cada uno me dara apoyo. Nadien esta esforzado a hacer algo que no quiera hacer. Esta reunion me dara una idea clara de en que puedo depender de ustedes. Tambien los ayudara si clarificamos la neturaleza de su apoyo para que esto no abrume a nadien.

Quiero repartir una lista de mis sintomas. Hay cosas que comienzan a pasarme cuando me comienzo a poner psicotico. Creo que es importante que esten enterados de esto porque cuando comienzo a poner me psicotico muchas veces yo no lo puedo ver. Si todos estedes comienzan a ver me haciendo estas cosas en la lista, como no comer, hablandome a mi mismo y pasando los dias en mi cuarto, ustedes saben que estoy en dificultad.

Guillo: ¿Que debemos hacer cuando te vemos asi?

Paciente: Bueno, el primer paso seria de hablarme de eso. Si te puedo oir, yo llamare a mi doctor para que me ayuda. Si encuentras que estoy incapaz de ayudarme a mi mismo, puedes llamar al numero de emergencia al final de la hoja. Ellos se responsabilisaran de ese punto en adelante—tu no tienes que hacer el trabajo de profesionales.

Incedentamente, yo firme formas de dar informacion para todos ustedes con mi terapista y mi psiquiatra. Esto significa que estan libres para hablar con ellos si necesitan, en una crisis, y ellos pudran dar les informacion.

Juan: ¿Entonces no tenemos que tratar de aconsejarte o nada? No es que no quiero ayudar, pero es que no sabria que hacer.

Paciente: ¡Estas correcto, Juan! Tu no debes de estar en esa posicion. Si necesitas ayuda profesional, llama a los profesionales y ellos se responsabilisaran.

¿Y tambien, hay otros sintomas o comportamientos que otros de ustedes ven cuando me enfermo que no puse en la lista?

Maria: Si, estaba persando que tu higiene es regularmente mala cuando te pones psicotico. No te afeitas ni te banas. Algunas veas tienes miedo de darte una ducha.

Paciente: Bien. Agregen lo a sus listas. ¿Algo mas?

(Silencio)

Bien. Vamos adelante a la lista de metodos en que me pueden dar apoyo. Las cosas que me pudieran aydara lo maximo seridan si pudiera tener una conversacion por telefono de diez al quinze minutos con alguien cuando estoy ansioso o solo y si alguien pudiera venir y cocinor y comer con migo cuando comienzo a decaer. Yo pare de comer las ultimas dos veces que fui hospitalizado. Creo que yo coneria si alguien estubiera con migo.

Maria: Yo vivo al labo de ti. Regularmente estoy por aqui a la hora de cenar. Esteria contenta de venir a cocinar y comer contigo. O, siguires, tu puedes venir y coner con nuestra familia.

Paciente: Gracias, Maria.

Guillo: Yo pudiera hablar contigo por telefono algunas veces. Tu sabes que trabajo horas largas y frequentemente no estoy en casa, pero cuando estoy estaria contento de hablar contigo si ayudaria.

Paciente: Gracias.

Juan: Si, tu me puedes llamar tambien. No me estorba.

Paciente: Gracias.

Jose: No se si supiera que decir si te estabas poniendo loco—no te ofendas.

Paciente: No te preocupes, Jose. Solo necesito que me asegures si estoy ansioso. O si me estoy aislando puedes sugerir que salga a ver a alguien o a hacer algo.

Jose: No se. Estoy un poco nervioso sobre esto.

Paciente: Esta bien Jose. No tienes que hacer esto si no estas comado.

Jose: Te llevaria a la sala de emergencia como la ultima vez si eso aydaria.

Paciente: Bueno. Eso fue algo que deveras me salvo la vida.

Jose: A la orden.

Maria: Solo dejanos saber que necesitas y ayudaremos si podemos.

Paciente: Muchas gracias. Entonces, Maria, Juan y Guillo estaran disponibles para hablar por telefono, Maria estara disponible para cenas y Jose me ayudara a llevarme a la sala de emergencia si lo necesito. Otra vez, deveras los aprecio a ustedes. Esto me significa mucho.

Hice torta y hay cafe. ¿Quien quiere?

HOSPITALIZATION REVIEW

The following worksheet is self-explanatory. It can be used in various ways. It can be assigned for homework and then discussed in a homework review. Alternatively, patients can work quietly through the first part of the group and then have a group discussion in the latter half of the group. Patients can work individually or in small groups.

This assignment assumes that you are working with people who have been psychiatrically hospitalized. If there are a number of people in the group who have not ever been hospitalized (highly unusual for an acute care day hospital program), run an alternative group for those who have not been hospitalized.

If someone has been hospitalized once, s/he obviously will not be able to see a pattern from one hospitalization to another; however, s/he may see a potential pattern and be able to take steps to avoid a second hospitalization. S/he will also benefit highly from listening to others discuss their experiences.

Worksheet
Hospitalization Review

In this exercise, you will examine your last three psychiatric hospitalizations. If you were hospitalized fewer than three times, just do as much as pertains to you.

Begin with your most recent psychiatric hospitalization. Answer the four questions for #1 about hospitalization. Take your time and think it through carefully. Then do the same with the questions in #2 for the previous hospitalization. After that, proceed with the questions in #3 for the first of the three hospitalizations.

1. a. Date of hospitalization _____

   b. Was anything stressful happening in your life right before you were hospitalized? If yes, describe:

   _____

   _____

   _____

   c. What were your symptoms?

   _____

   _____

   _____

   d. For how long were you having these symptoms before you went into the hospital?

   _____

   e. How did you handle the period of time between the onset of your symptoms and your hospitalization?

   _____

   _____

   _____

   _____

f. If you could go back to that time today, what would you do differently, if anything?

_____

_____

_____

2. a. Date of hospitalization _____

b. Was anything stressful happening in your life right before you were hospitalized? If yes, describe:

_____

_____

_____

_____

c. What were your symptoms?

_____

_____

_____

d. For how long were you having these symptoms before you went into the hospital?

_____

e. How did you handle the period of time between the onset of your symptoms and your hospitalization?

_____

_____

_____

_____

f. If you could go back to that time today, what would you do differently, if anything?

_____

_____

_____

_____

3. a. Date of hospitalization _____

b. Was anything stressful happening in your life right before you were hospitalized? If yes, describe:

_____

_____

_____

_____

c. What were your symptoms?

_____

_____

_____

d. For how long were you having these symptoms before you went into the hospital?

_____

e. How did you handle the period of time between the onset of your symptoms and your hospitalization?

_____

_____

_____

f. If you could go back to that time today, what would you do differently, if anything?

_____

_____

_____

_____

Is there any pattern to the dates of your hospitalizations? For example, do they all occur at approximately the same time of the year? Do they occur around the anniversary of some event in your life?

_____

_____

_____

Do you see any similarities in 1b, 2b, and 3b? If so, describe:

_____

_____

_____

Did you have any difficulty identifying your symptoms? Did you have difficulty identifying them at the time they occurred? Could you be on the lookout for them in the future?

_____

_____

_____

What observations can you make about questions e and f for all three hospitalizations? How will these observations help you in avoiding a future hospitalization?

_____

_____

_____

_____

Repaso De Hospitalizacion

En este ejercicio vas a examinar tus ultimas tres hospitalizaciones psiquiatricas. Si fuistes hospitalizado menos de tres veces solamente haz lo que te corresponde.

Comienza con tu hospitalizacion psiquiatrica mas reciente. Contesta las quatro preguntas para el #1 sobre esa hospitalizacion. Toma tu tiempo y piensalo muy bien. Despues, haz lo mismo con las preguntas en el #2 para la penultima hospitalizacion. Despues de eso, sigue con las preguntas en el #3 para la primera de las tres hospitalizacions.

1. a. Fecha de hospitalizacion _____

   b. ¿Habia algo causandote tension en tu vida immediatamente antes de que fuistes hospitalizado? Si tu respuesta es "si," describe:

      _____

      _____

      _____

   c. ¿Cuales eran tus sintomas?

      _____

      _____

      _____

   d. ¿Por cuanto tiempo estabas teniendo estos sintomas antes de entrar al hospital?

      _____

   e. ¿Como manejastes este peniodo de tiempo entre cuando comenzaron los sintomas y cuando te hospitalizastes?

      _____

      _____

      _____

f. ¿Si pudieras regresar a ese periodo de tiempo hoy, que harias diferentemente, si hay algo?

_____

_____

_____

2. a. Fecha de hospitalizacion _____

b. ¿Habia algo causandote tension en tu vida immediatamente antes de que fuistes hospitalizado? Si tu respuesta es "si," describe:

_____

_____

_____

_____

c. ¿Cuales eran tus sintomas?

_____

_____

_____

d. ¿Por cuanto tiempo estabas teniendo estos sintomas antes de entrar al hospital?

_____

e. ¿Como manejastes este peniodo de tiempo entre cuando comenzaron los sintomas y cuando te hospitalizastes?

_____

_____

_____

f. ¿Si pudieras regresar a ese periodo de tiempo hoy, que harias diferentemente, si hay algo?

_____

_____

_____

_____

3. a. Fecha de hospitalizacion _____

b. ¿Habia algo causandote tension en tu vida immediatamente antes de que fuistes hospitalizado? Si tu respuesta es "si," describe:

_____

_____

_____

_____

c. ¿Cuales eran tus sintomas?

_____

_____

_____

d. ¿Por cuanto tiempo estabas teniendo estos sintomas antes de entrar al hospital?

_____

e. ¿Como manejastes este peniodo de tiempo entre cuando comenzaron los sintomas y cuando te hospitalizastes?

_____

_____

_____

_____

f. ¿Si pudieras regresar a ese periodo de tiempo hoy, que harias diferentemente, si hay algo?

_____

_____

_____

_____

¿Hay alguna norma de las fechas de tus hospitalizaciones? ¿Por ejemplo, ocurren todas aproximadamente al mismo tiempo del ano? ¿Ocurren al rededor del aniversario de algun evento en tu vida?

_____

_____

_____

¿Vez algunas senejanzas entre 1b, 2b, y 3b? Si hay, describe:

_____

_____

_____

¿Tienes alguna dificultad identificando tus sintomas? ¿Tuvistes dificultad identificando los durante el tiempo que estaban occuriendo? ¿Pudieras estar preparado para reconocer los en el futoro?

_____

_____

_____

¿Cuales observaciones puedes hacer sobre las preguntas e y f por todas tres hospitalizaciones? ¿Como te ayudaran estas observaciones en previniendo una hospitalizacion en el futuro?

_____

_____

_____

_____

WHAT'S IN A HOSPITAL?

Preparation

None!

Activity

Begin by having patients list things they did not like about being in a (psychiatric) hospital. Write the list on the board. This can be used as an incentive to stay out of the hospital. Discuss these items with that goal in mind. Typical answers include: being locked in, having to get up at a certain time, loss of freedom, the food, etc.

Erase the board. Next have patients list what they liked about the hospital. This list should go down the left side of the board only. Leave space underneath each item. You may need more than one board. On the right side, have patients list ways that they could achieve each of those items *without* going into the hospital. For example, an item on the list might be, "I got away from my children for a week." Ask the patients how they can get away from their children for a week without being hospitalized.

In some cases the list of what people liked about the hospital is considerably longer than the list of what people didn't like about the hospital. If this happens, point it out and have a discussion about their feelings concerning hospitalization.

CRISIS GAME

Preparation

All you need are the questions that follow.

Activity

Divide the group into two or three teams. Have one person on each team be the writer, for which a notebook and pen are needed.

You will read one of the crisis items. The groups will then have two minutes to come up with as many different solutions as possible. They should speak softly to one another so they don't give answers away to their opposing teams. At the end of two minutes, the teams will announce their answers. The team with the most legitimate answers wins the point.

This group works best if you can be a little outrageous and run it like a game show with you playing the role of a game show host. It might lift your own spirits if you're having a rough day.

CRISES

1. You take the van to the day hospital. You realize afterward that you might have left the stove on. No one else lives with you. What do you do?
2. Your pet gets sick in the middle of the night. You have no transportation. What do you do?
3. You have a college exam. You have been very depressed and you're completely unprepared. What do you do?
4. You are not a U.S. citizen. Your visa will run out in two weeks. You have an important exam to take in six weeks. What do you do?
5. You bought a used car from a car dealership. It's been rigged, and it completely breaks down two days later. The dealership will not refund your money. What do you do?
6. Your disability check will be late because of a computer error. Your rent is due and you don't have the money. What do you do?
7. You have to move to a new apartment. You have no money for the security. What do you do?
8. Your landlord notifies you that he is selling the house. You must be out in thirty days. What do you do?
9. You are an alcoholic. You have the strong urge to take a drink. What do you do?
10. Your doctor changed your medication. You forgot to fill the prescription and it's too late to go to the drugstore. What do you do?
11. Your car breaks down. It's the only car you have. You have to get to work. What do you do?
12. The phone company sends you a shut-off notice. What do you do?
13. You lose your job. Jobs are hard to find in your field and you haven't saved any money. What do you do?
14. You lose all your keys. What do you do?
15. Someone snatches your purse. What do you do?
16. Someone hits your car on the highway and tries to get away. You can see them close by. What do you do?

17. Your daughter has no place to live. She asks to live with you. You really don't want her to live with you. What do you do?
18. You are bipolar. You're very excited on your birthday. You're not sure if you're having a mild manic episode. What do you do?
19. You need emergency housing. The only housing you can find won't allow you to have your two cats with whom you have lived for seven years. You are unwilling to put them in a shelter. What do you do?
20. You find out that your spouse is having an affair. What do you do?
21. You discover that your roommate is using cocaine. What do you do?

SAMPLE: CRISIS GAME

Question: Your pet gets sick in the middle of the night. You
                 have no transportation. What do you do?

Answers

Team A: Take a taxi.

                 Call a neighbor for a ride.

                 Call your parents for a ride.

                 Make the pet comfortable and take a bus first thing
                 in the morning.

Answers

Team B: Stay calm. Pray to your highest power.

                 Take a taxi.

                 Get a friend to take you to an emergency clinic.

Team A would get the point with four answers. Notice that Team
B's first answer might be considered controversial. How do you
decide which answers to accept and which ones to reject? The rule
of thumb is that you should accept answers that do no harm, address
the situation, and/or help the patient. For those in recovery, talking
to their highest power may be key during a crisis.

A NOTE ABOUT SKITS

Following are two ways in which skits can be used therapeutically. Hopefully you will invent others as well.

One thing you need to remember about skits is that, while you may be fantasizing about a Broadway production, you will be working with people whose affect is flat, who are anhedonic and withdrawn, and who may even have trouble reading. The first time I did the conflict resolution skit, I almost burst out laughing *at myself* when I heard a group of people slowly and flatly repeat the words on the page. They often didn't even notice when it was their turn to speak and had to be cued. This wasn't what I had in mind and, at first, it wasn't much fun. Once they got warmed up, however, and once I involved some of the higher-functioning patients (that first group didn't include any) things improved. And once I got in on the scene and added some melodrama of my own, it got a lot better. Melodrama can be helpful in "waking people up." After I pretended to throw a major temper tantrum in one of the skits and ended by throwing my papers across the room, several people with waxy stares came to life.

The crisis skit works better when you have a number of higher-functioning patients, meaning patients with some creativity who are somewhat expressive and have the capacity to write a script. You can include lower-functioning people but the higher-functioning people need to take the lead. The conflict resolution skit (see Chapter 8) works better for a lower-functioning group because half the lines are written for them. Also there are not the components of the props, costumes, etc.

Skits are wonderful for helping people to open up—to communicate about things they might not otherwise share. I will never forget the time when one very sullen patient came to our day hospital. All she talked about for days was how much she didn't want to be there. She had a very gloomy look on her face constantly. When we did the crisis skit, she wrote the skit. She played the part of an alcoholic father who terrorized the family. A man played the part of a spineless wife with a high-pitched voice and the two fought bitterly. Others played the parts of intimidated children. The skit was done as a comedy and it was so funny that we were all holding our stomachs laughing. When it was over, after acknowledging the players, we had a serious discussion about alcoholic family systems. The patient was engaged in treatment from that point on.

CRISIS SKIT

Preparation

You might want to add to the skit by providing all kinds of materials from which costumes and props could be made. This could include cloth, paper, old clothes, jewelry (if you are working with suicidal people, be careful of sharp objects or belts), tape recordings of sounds or music, artistic materials from which a back-drop could be made, etc.

Activity

Divide the patients into groups of approximately five. Have them write a skit in which they will depict a crisis and its resolution. Make sure when you create the groups that you evenly divide the higher-functioning patients who might have a greater capacity for creativity, reading, and writing, and the lower-functioning patients who might not be able to contribute a great deal to the creative process and might only be able to handle having one line in the skit.

Have the patients create props and costumes for the skit. These do not have to be elaborate. They can note items they need that are not available and discuss ways of providing them for the next day when the skits will be performed. The props could include sound effects, smells, backdrops, costumes, and so forth. Emphasize that they should have fun and be creative without feeling pressured to make this into a Broadway production.

The skits should be performed later that day or the next day, as seems best to you. I do not recommend performing them more than twenty-four hours later if you are working in a short-term day hospital setting because, in my experience, the change of clientele is sufficient to ruin a team's work in just a few days.

Discussion

Have everyone discuss the crisis and its resolution after each performance. Were other resolutions possible? Was the one proposed a feasible one? How many others have faced the crisis in question?

Additional Questions

Address the following questions to the patients to stimulate further discussion:

What minor "crises" did you face in preparing this skit? How did you think through the problems? Were they successfully resolved? How did you feel when the crises occurred? How did you feel while resolving them?

What crises do you dread facing? Why? How might these be resolved?

Chapter 5

Goal Setting and Support

Day hospital programming is extremely challenging. Most of the programming involves the use of groups. You are sometimes required to justify *each* patient's involvement in each group by discussing the relationship between that patient's treatment plan objectives and the content of the group. Since everyone's treatment plan is different, this is a very tall order. Groups that have goal setting as a focus help the patients relate their work in the day hospital directly to their treatment plans.

Without a structure for support, goal setting is reduced to just that. Patients set the goals and then forget about them, much the way people make New Year's resolutions and then forget about them. It is the structure for support that keeps the goals fresh in the patients' minds.

Structure for support can take various forms. Patients can check in with each other every day when they see each other in the day hospital. They might call each other at home if that is appropriate. For example, a patient who promises to get up no later than 10:00 a.m. on both Saturday and Sunday might require a phone call from a support buddy on both of those days to make sure that s/he is up. Support may take other creative forms as well. One obese patient agreed to stick with her diet for the week. Three other patients sat with her in the cafeteria each day to support her in staying away from the junk food. Some withdrawn patients set a goal of saying one thing in group every day. Their buddies agreed to poke them in the ribs if they haven't said anything and the group is about to draw to a close. Some patients set a goal of staying awake in groups. Their buddies also poke them in the ribs—when they fall asleep. Buddies have also accompanied patients to AA, NA, or Al-Anon meetings.

The Five-Day Project Creation/Review occurs weekly first thing Monday morning (creation) and last thing on Friday (review). Recently I have experimented with having patients check off goals as they accomplish them throughout the week. The goals are written on a large sheet of paper that is hung on the wall in the day room. This keeps the goals fresh in their minds and allows them to end the day with a sense of accomplishment as I make this part of a wrap-up meeting at the end of the day.

The Mountain Exercise helps people with long-term goal setting. This exercise is difficult for patients. I have found that they have difficulty partializing and also making goals concrete and measurable. They tend to cringe when asked to set target dates for goals. It is useful to discuss how to relate to missing a target; many patients tend to beat themselves up over this.

FIVE-DAY PROJECT CREATION/REVIEW

This extremely simple group ensures that treatment plan objectives are being actively pursued. The clinician uses the treatment plan to help the patient set goals for the week.

Preparation

Hang a large sheet of paper on the wall and have markers ready. Also, bring a copy of everyone's treatment plan to the group meeting.

Activity

The first group on Monday should be Five-Day Project Creation. Each person decides on at least one goal to pursue for the week. The goal should be concrete and measurable. Some patients may have more than one goal. No one should have more than three.

Patients will share their goals with the group. Write the goals on the sheet of paper. If any goals are unrealistic or unrelated to the treatment plan, the clinician should help the patient redefine them.

Next to each person's goals, write the name of someone in the room who will support the person during the week. Everyone should have at least one person to support. Support can take various forms—a gentle reminder of a goal during groups, a phone call at home, checking in with the person during breaks or during lunch, etc.

Also, everyone on staff should be aware of each person's goals. Patients should be encouraged to discuss their goals with their social workers and psychiatrists. Staff should be encouraged to raise the topic during weekly meetings.

The last group on Friday is Five-Day Project Review. During this group, people review their progress with their goals and gain some closure on that week's project. A weekend goal may be set if desired.

SAMPLE: FIVE DAY PROJECT CREATION
Week of July 5–July 9, 1999

Who	Goal	Support
Mary	1. Do all laundry on Wednesday without help.	John
	2. Call friend and make plans for weekend social activity.	
Joe	1. Will speak once in every group.	Hilda
Clyde	1. Will meet with support team.	Mary
	2. Will apply for one job.	
	Etc. . . .	

THE MOUNTAIN EXERCISE

Preparation

For this group you will need copies of the Mountain Exercise Sheet (see Figure 5.1). This exercise should be done in pencil as it may require many erasures; have them available.

Introductory Remarks

Imagine that you are about to go on a mountain climbing expedition. You have your gear. You look up to the top of a high mountain. You can barely see it. You have your doubts, but taking a deep breath, you bend your knees and jump as high as you can. When you see that you did not make it to the top you try again. After a third try you give up in despair.

This is the way we approach many of our goals. Instead of mapping them out step by step, we simply "go for it." When we don't achieve those goals with one attempt, we belittle ourselves and give up, blame someone else, and/or continue trying what doesn't work.

This exercise is about mapping out your proverbial mountain climb. It is about taking a goal and dividing it into subgoals and even sub-subgoals. It's about taking that journey one step at a time and being fully aware of each step.

Activity

Begin by asking each patient to establish a goal. This goal will be written on the top right side of the page next to the word *Goal.* Before writing the goal, each goal should be stated out loud so that you can help the patient to refine it if necessary. Revision will be needed for goals that are unrealistic, too small, or poorly defined (e.g., "to feel better"). It is especially important that goals be concrete and measurable ("to obtain my bachelor's degree by May 1999").

Next explain that the person on the bottom left corner of the page is beginning a journey up the mountain, step by step, toward the fulfillment of the goal. The person begins by establishing a first subgoal. This subgoal, listed on the left, will then be further divided into sub-subgoals. The sub-subgoals are a list of steps necessary to achieve the subgoal. For example, the first subgoal for the person who wants to complete a bachelor's degree by May 1999 might be to "get stable and remain stable." Sub-subgoals might include "find the right medication and take it regularly," "find a therapist," "get ongoing support from others with my illness," "learn to recognize the first signs that I am getting sick." The righthand side of the page is the "By when?" side. It answers the question, "By when will this subgoal be accomplished?" The date should be specific, including at least a month and year.

Continue in this way all the way up the mountain. It is not necessary that there be five subgoals. If there are more than five subgoals, the patient can make his or her own sheet with spaces for the proper number of goals.

The sheet should be posted in a place where the patient will view it frequently (e.g., refrigerator door) and use it as a reference and encouragement.

A word of caution: Make sure the patients choose goals to which they are genuinely committed.

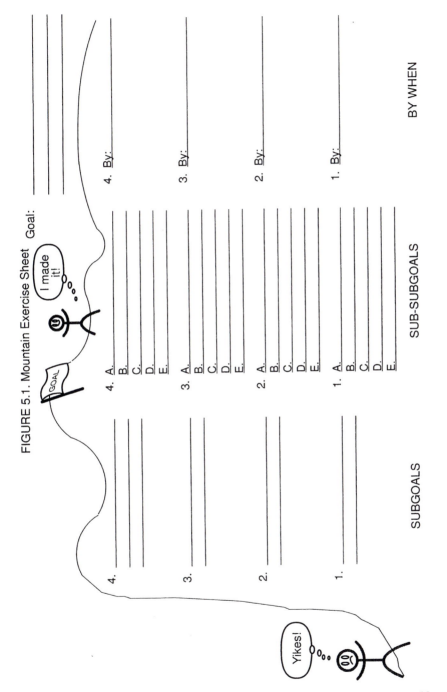

FIGURE 5.1. Mountain Exercise Sheet

BELMONT UNIVERSITY LIBRARY

FIGURE 5.1. (continued)

Goal: Have my own apartment by December 1999

SUBGOALS	SUB-SUBGOALS	BY WHEN
4. Obtain apartment	4. A. Save money for security B. Save money for rent C. Look at apartments D. Sign a lease E.	4. By: December 1, 1999
3. Brush up on ADLs	3. A. Do more cooking at home B. Do laundry and ironing C. Make list of potential crises & learn to solve D. Open & maintain bank account E. Do food shopping	3. By: October 31, 1999
2. Find a job that pays enough for an apartment	2. A. Construct resumé B. Search classifieds C. Go to places and apply D. Brush up on job interview skills E. Buy work clothes	2. By: October 31, 1999
1. Get stabilized and stay stabilized	1. A. Follow medication regimen B. Find a therapist & begin therapy C. Find a private psychiatrist D. E.	1. By: September 15, 1999

Chapter 6

Cognitive Restructuring

Cognitive restructuring is excellent for people with depression or anxiety. It is also a useful way to help patients with other disorders, such as schizophrenia, to attack disempowering assumptions that they may make about their futures. For example, many patients believe that they will undoubtedly end up in the hospital again. Some believe that they will never be able to work because they have lost many jobs in the past, even though they may be much healthier today than they were at that time.

There are some terrific books that help patients in this area and from which you can derive groups. A couple of examples include *The Depression Workbook* by Mary Ellen Copeland, *The Anxiety and Phobia Workbook* by Edmund J. Bourne and *The Relaxation Workbook* by Martha Davis, Elizabeth R. Eshelman, and Matthew McKay (see bibliography for details).

This chapter includes a few innovative groups for cognitive restructuring. The modality involved is the use of metaphor. In Shades of Gray . . . and More: Exploding Dichotomous Thinking, color is used as a metaphor to illustrate the limitations of dichotomous thinking (or black-and-white thinking). Not only is the group fun, but the metaphor helps patients to understand an abstract psychological concept.

The Blue Car Syndrome illustrates the concept of overgeneralizing with a ridiculous story. Exaggeration is a great way to teach an abstract concept.

I designed Singing in the Rain: From Adversity to Advantage to illustrate fatalistic thinking. This group helps patients to understand the element of interpretation in what we see. This is accomplished by having the patients create various unconventional uses for conventional objects such as a pencil and a tuning fork. I also include the story of Puddleglum, a character in one of C.S. Lewis's stories whose thinking is extremely negative. The homework may be done as part of the group (individually or in small groups) or at home. If it is done at home, it should be reviewed at a later time.

Murphy's Law Revisited is another group that allows patients to change their cognitive constructs. We seldom laugh at our own ridiculous thoughts. We do laugh at Murphy's Laws, however. Helping the patients frame their disempowering thoughts as personal "Murphy's Laws" allows them to see these negative thoughts in a new light. It also allows them to lighten up!

SHADES OF GRAY ... AND MORE:
EXPLODING DICHOTOMOUS THINKING

Preparation

Set up a card table with objects of various colors. Include as many colors as you possibly can. Arrange the table to be as attractive as possible. Make sure a black object and a white object are included. Have a tablecloth or large piece of white paper covering the objects on the table when the group begins. Have a separate pile of other objects, as discussed below.

Activity

Using objects from the pile (the table is still covered), hold up an object that is black. Ask what the color is. Then hold up a white object. Ask what color it is. Next hold up something that is dark gray and ask for the color. Then hold up something light gray. (The group will probably distinguish between dark and light gray.) Next hold up a series of three objects that are different shades of the same color, such as dark green, mint green, and kelly green. Point out that they are all green. Discuss the difficulty we would have if we had no way of distinguishing one "green" from another.

Now uncover the table. Have people get up and look closely at the table. Have them comment on the various colors and shades of colors. The table should include objects of more than one color as well as objects of various shapes. Ask the patients how many colors they see on the table. Ask them how many colors they think exist in the universe. Hopefully this will lead to some debate. Allow the debate to go on for a bit. If no one has, suggest the possibility that an infinite number of colors exists in the universe.

Now take the black object and the white object off the table and re-cover the table. Hold these objects up. Ask, "What if these were the only two colors you knew about? How would you fare as an artist? How would the world look to you?"

Compare this situation to "black-and-white thinking." Some examples of black-and-white (dichotomous) thinking include:

It has to be perfect or it's no good.

If I don't have a car, I can't get anywhere.

If my husband leaves me, I'll be lost.

Point out that each of these cognitions carries with it only two possibilities, one of which leads to total despair.

Have patients write down examples of black-and-white thoughts that they have. Then have others in the group generate the "shades of gray," the other alternatives. Do this once or twice with the whole group. Then either have the patients work individually or in small groups. Toward the end, regather as a whole group to share. You might like to have one or two people write their examples on the board for group discussion.

SAMPLE

Black-and-White Thought: If I don't get a car, I won't be able to get a job.

Two Possibilities from This Thought:

1. I get a car and get a job.
2. I don't get a car and therefore have no job (the "no-possibility" possibility).

Alternatives:

1. I use public transportation, limiting my job search to places I can get to by bus or train.
2. I move to New York City.
3. I get a ride from someone.
4. I get a job within walking distance from my home.
5. I work out of my home.

Worksheet

SHADES OF GRAY . . . AND MORE: EXPLODING DICHOTOMOUS THINKING

Black-and-White Thought:

Two Possibilities from This Thought:

 1.
 2.

Alternatives:

Black-and-White Thought:

Two Possibilities from This Thought:

 1.
 2.

Alternatives:

Black-and-White Thought:

Two Possibilities from This Thought:

 1.
 2.

Alternatives:

THE BLUE CAR SYNDROME

Preparation

None!

Activity

Read the following short story:

> Yesterday I saw an accident on the way to work. A blue car ran into another car. The accident was clearly the fault of the driver in the blue car. Today as I was driving to work, I carefully avoided all blue cars. When I saw a blue car behind me, I switched lanes on the highway. I kept a good distance away from the blue car in front of me. I had to keep jogging back and forth to avoid these cars—I've never seen so many blue cars in my life! Some of them were a blueish or greenish color and it was hard to tell if they were blue, so I avoided them to be on the safe side. I was about to get on one road, but I saw a number of blue cars so I took another road instead. Actually, now I try to travel on off hours when traffic is light in the hopes of running into less of these cars.

Discuss the problem of this story with the patients. Introduce the notion of overgeneralization.

Have the patients write their own ridiculous stories to demonstrate overgeneralization. This should add a few good laughs to the group.

Discuss the following:

1. What is the effect of overgeneralizing?
2. In what ways do you overgeneralize?
3. What price have you paid for this?

Homework

Instruct the patients to pay attention to the way they overgeneralize for the next week. When they notice an overgeneralization, they should jot down the statement and correct it. For example:

Error: Everything is going wrong today.
Correction: Two things went wrong this morning.

SINGING IN THE RAIN:
FROM ADVERSITY TO ADVANTAGE

Preparation

Have handy a pair of high-heeled shoes, a pencil, and a tool with which most people would be unfamiliar, such as a tuning fork. You might also like to use the references from C.S. Lewis's *Chronicles of Narnia* mentioned below. If you choose to read these, you might want to make copies for everyone in order to aid those who have difficulty following along because of poor concentration skills.

Activity 1

Hold up a pair of high-heeled shoes and ask the group what they see. Hopefully they will say "shoes." Tell them that you also see a triangle and hold the shoes together by placing the heels and the soles together as in the illustration below.

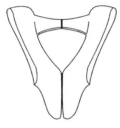

Hold up a pencil. Ask the group what they see. They'll be more creative this time. Some examples might include a conductor's baton, a back scratcher, a straight edge, and a weapon.

Hold up a tool with which people are usually unfamiliar, such as a tuning fork for a piano. Ask them what they see.

Questions for Discussion

1. If we see such variety in concrete things, is it any wonder that we see other things differently?
2. Why is it that, when you go to court, there are at least two different versions of the story? Is it just because people are purposely lying? Is it that they remember things differently? Why do we remember things differently?

3. How does all this relate to negative thinking? When people are thinking negatively, is it because negative things are happening or because they see the things that are happening negatively?

Activity 2

Read pages 58 through 64 (in Chapter 5) of *The Silver Chair* by C.S. Lewis (C.S. Lewis, *The Silver Chair*. New York: Macmillan Publishing Company, 1953). This section is about a creature named Puddleglum whose thinking is extremely negative.

Questions for Discussion

1. Do you think that, if it rains, the weather is bad? What is bad about rain? What is good about rain?

Some Possible Answers:	It's fun to play in puddles, it fills reservoirs, waters plants and keeps umbrella manufacturers in business.

2. Is it bad to lose your job? What good could come from losing your job?

Some Possible Answers:	You could get a better job, you could rest, collect unemployment, and appreciate your next job all the more.

Activity 3

Explain to the patients the notion of "fatalistic thinking." Have them write in their notebooks examples of fatalistic thinking in their own lives. List some of these examples on the board. Examples might include the following:

Nothing ever goes right for me.

I know that I'm going to end up back in the hospital.

I'm never going to get a job (get married, etc.).

Nobody likes me.

Correct these statements to reflect facts only. Example:

"Nothing ever goes right for me" can be corrected to state, "In the past, some difficult things have happened. That has nothing to do with now."

Homework

List fatalistic thoughts and corresponding corrections from your own life. If possible, use examples from your present life, not the past.

1. Fatalistic Thought

Correction

2. Fatalistic Thought

Correction

3. Fatalistic Thought

Correction

MURPHY'S LAW REVISITED

Preparation

Hang several large sheets of paper on the wall. Have markers handy.

Activity

Remind the group of Murphy's Law: "If anything can go wrong, it will."

Discuss a few examples of Murphy's Law. They can either be "laws" that you read somewhere or ones that you make up. Begin with impersonal ones such as:

- It always rains when you plan a picnic.
- The movie you wanted to see always leaves the theatre right before you have time to see it.
- The phone call you didn't want to miss comes when you are in the bathroom.

Allow this to be a time of "lightening up." Make this fun.

Have the group eventually begin to name the personal "Murphy's Laws" that they encounter. These should be written on the large sheets of paper in one color. Space should be left underneath each one for writing a correction in another color. Examples might include:

- Whenever I try to get a job, I don't get it.
- Whenever I get into a relationship, I mess it up.
- Whenever I try to make friends, they leave me.

When the group has written down their "laws," add the corrections using another color. Have them look at what actually happened that led them to make that law. For example:

• Whenever I try to get a job, I don't get it.

I went on two job interviews and didn't get the jobs.

• Whenever I try to make friends, they leave me.

My four friends all left me when I had a psychotic episode and entered the hospital. Now I am not psychotic.

Chapter 7

Activities of Daily Living

Because this area is emphasized in many programs, I do not feel the need to elaborate too much on this therapeutic theme. One activity frequently used in day hospitals is cooking. The problem with cooking groups is they sometimes degenerate into recreation (or simply mundane activity) rather than therapeutic activity. The key here, as with all activities, is to make the therapeutic goal paramount and to tailor the milieu in such a way that it *serves* the therapeutic goal. In this day and age, however, we must refer to therapeutic *goals* because, as I mentioned earlier, some managed care companies now expect us to relate each patient's participation in the group to his or her specific treatment plan. How, then, can you tailor a cooking group (or any other activity) to meet multiple, individual goals? And what should those goals be?

Cooking and Nutrition discusses this very issue. Just for fun, I include a little game called, "What If . . . " that you can play with the patients while waiting for things to cook in the oven or on the stove. The game addresses everyday problems related to cooking.

I also include a few comments about simulation of activities of daily living.

The Balancing Act is an example of a simulation invented for the day hospital program. The design work is time-consuming originally, but it then can be used numerous times.

COOKING AND NUTRITION

Day hospital programs often use cooking as an activity, especially since a kitchen is often one of the facilities available to the day hospital staff. Cooking groups, however, have a tendency to be recreational rather than therapeutic. This section will help you design your cooking activities so that they are therapeutic and aligned with the expectations of managed care companies.

Keep two things in mind: activities should in some way relate to the abatement of symptoms being targeted for treatment, and activities may address activities of daily living. It is important, however, to address those activities of daily living that are genuinely a problem for each patient. If the patient already knows how to cook, it will be difficult to justify putting him or her in a cooking class.

Let's look at a few symptoms that you may address in the milieu. You may address these whether or not the individual knows how to cook.

Akathisia	Is this person able to stand/sit still to perform a task, or must s/he constantly get up to pace back and forth? Can you use the activity to try to decrease the amount of pacing?
Amotivation	What initiative do you see when introducing the cooking tasks? Is this someone who must be told every last thing to do? Is s/he sitting or sleeping on the side while others are working? Does s/he ask to do anything?
Autonomy/ Dependence	Can this person work autonomously or does s/he helplessly back out of tasks, consistently and unnecessarily enlisting the aid of others?
Concentration	Can this person attend to a task from beginning to end? For what span of time can s/he concentrate?
Energy Level	Is this person heavily sedated? Does s/he possess sufficient energy to carry out simple tasks?
Gross and Fine Motor Skills	Can this person hold a knife and cut something? Can s/he break an egg into a dish? Or are his or her hands shaking too much?

Impulsivity	Does this person follow directions or impulsively do things on her or his own? Does s/he rush through tasks too quickly, doing a poor job? Does s/he move tangentially from one task to another without finishing anything? Is speech pressured? Is s/he irritable? Can s/he be redirected when necessary?
Internal Preoccupation	Is this person preoccupied with internal stimuli? Is s/he aware of what is occurring in the environment?
Judgment	How do you rate this person's judgment with regard to how high to have the flame, what to do if something isn't boiling after a long time, how large to cut the vegetables, when to start cooking various items, etc.?
Memory	Is this person able to remember instructions? If not, is s/he able to compensate with written instructions to which s/he can frequently refer?
Problem Solving	Is this person able to generate creative solutions to miniature crises that occur in the kitchen (e.g., discovering that s/he doesn't have a necessary ingredient, something is boiling over or burning, etc.)?
Social Functioning	How does this person interact with others? Is his/her social functioning adequate for autonomous living in the community?

These are some examples of issues that can be addressed in the cooking groups. *The key is to center the tasks around these therapeutic issues* rather than centering the tasks around what is necessary to most efficiently cook the meal.

It is also possible to utilize the cooking groups to address problems with activities of daily living. *The key is to assess the needs of each patient so that you can tailor your activities to those needs.*

There are two ways to assess the patients' skills. One is to do a written and/or oral interview. The other is to observe them during their first cooking group, asking them to perform various tasks. You can record observations in a progress note. Following are hypothetical examples.

HYPOTHETICAL INTERVIEW

How many meals do you eat on an average day?

What do you usually eat—for breakfast?

   —for lunch?

   —for dinner?

How many times a week, on average, do you eat out?

Who usually does the cooking in your home?

If you do not now live on your own, do you anticipate living on your own in the future? If so, when?

What items are you able to cook now?

What items would you like to be able to cook?

Do you have access to a kitchen? If no, do you have a hot plate or a rice cooker?

What are your biggest problems in the areas of food shopping, cooking, and eating?

Plan for further assessment:

Treatment Plan:

_____   _____
Signature of Staff   Signature of Patient

_____   _____
Date   Date

HYPOTHETICAL PROGRESS NOTE FROM OBSERVATION

Patient Name: John Doe
Case No.:   000-00-0000
Date: 1/1/2001
Unit: Adult Day Hospital

John Doe participated in his first cooking group today. He experiences chronic auditory hallucinations and is often internally preoccupied. He lives in a boarding home.

John reported that he often skips meals because he runs out of money. He does not cook. He usually eats at Burger King or McDonald's or the local diner. He continues this until the third week of the month when his money typically runs out. He then relies on the local soup kitchen for one meal per day. It is noteworthy that John weighs 320 pounds and suffers from sleep apnea.

John began the cooking group by going to the couch in the corner of the room and falling asleep. When asked to participate, he was reluctant at first but eventually agreed. He was asked to read a part of the recipe (minestrone soup) and determine which cooking utensils were needed. He was able to identify most of the utensils and lay them out on the counter. There were no problems with fine or gross motor skills.

John was asked to read a part of the recipe and determine what needed to be done. He was able to do this accurately. He had little difficulty peeling potatoes. He was also asked to work at the stove (placed pot of water on the stove and boiled). He exercised reasonable judgment at the stove.

Assessment: John possesses the capacity to learn some cooking skills. While in the day hospital, the goal will be to teach him to cook three nutritious, inexpensive meals that don't require a stove. Emphasis will be placed on helping John to stretch his budget so that he can eat throughout the entire month. John will also learn the basics of nutrition and be counseled in choosing more appropriate foods at the diner.

What If . . . ?

1. What if you are making soup and you burn it?
2. What if you realize partway through your cooking that you ran out of milk?
3. What if a box was too close to the flame and caught on fire?
4. What if the electricity went off and you had a lot of food in the refrigerator?
5. What if you ran out of food and you had no money?
6. What if you noticed that, every time you use the oven, your food is undercooked?
7. What if a casserole boiled over in the oven and left a huge mess in it that started to smoke up the house?
8. What if you got an important phone call while you were cooking eggs?
9. What if you wanted toast and found out that the toaster didn't work?
10. What if you got very depressed and didn't have the energy to cook?
11. What if the buses weren't running and you had to get to the grocery store?
12. What if the recipe called for a garlic press and you didn't have one?
13. What if you lived someplace where you didn't have a stove?
14. What if you finished cooking rice and found out it was still hard?
15. What if you burned your hand badly on a pot?
16. What if you had a coupon for an item and discovered the store had no more of that item on the shelf?
17. What if you had to cook a large meal for company and started to feel overwhelmed?
18. What if the top of the salt shaker fell off while you were pouring salt into the pot, causing you to pour a huge amount of salt into the food?

SIMULATION FOR ACTIVITIES OF DAILY LIVING

Initial assessments should include assessment of the patients' deficits in activities of daily living. These may include cooking, cleaning, laundry, bathing, shaving, budgeting, using a checking account, ironing, paying bills, clothes shopping, getting out of bed in the morning, taking medications independently at home, and so on.

Activities of daily living are best learned by simulation (a type of role rehearsal) and then by practice at home. For example, if there are patients who do not know how to do laundry, the day hospital might organize a trip to the laundromat. Rags could be used instead of clothes. These rags might have various stains on them to demonstrate the various skills needed to handle the stains. Patients should be talked through the process at the laundromat. *They* should be the ones sorting the laundry, putting in the detergent, etc. Written instructions should accompany the lesson. These instructions should be included in the patients' notebooks.

After this, during the Five-Day Project Creation group on Monday morning, the patients should set a weekly goal of doing their own laundry. They should choose a day to do it and follow through with their caseworkers the next day.

People who are not bathing might be sent to the shower, if there is one in the facility, with soap and a towel. People requiring help with shaving might have a private lesson in the men's room with shaving cream and a razor provided by the staff (be sure to take the razor back when the lesson is over!). Other items that should be handy are combs, shampoo, soap, towels, a hair dryer, an iron, an ironing board, rags, laundry detergent, stain removers, petty cash for washing machines and dryers, cleanser, window cleaner, dust remover, a vacuum, broom, mop, bucket, floor cleaner, other cleaning items, an alarm clock (for demonstration), and pill boxes (the inexpensive plastic type).

Following is a simulation group designed to help people learn how to use a checking account. A similar group could be designed to teach people how to pay bills.

THE BALANCING ACT

Preparation

This group involves a lot of preparation the first time you do it, but it is worth it. It's easier after that.

Obtain as many blank check registers as you can from a local bank—as a donation, if possible.

Create a series of twenty checks drawn from an account with "Day Hospital Savings and Loan Association." If you wish, you may use the sample (see Figure 7.1). Make many copies of the blank checks.

Make up a list of people to whom the checks should be made out along with the amounts (see Table 7.1). Make plenty of copies.

Now make out a statement (see Table 7.2). Make copies.

Activity

Patients are first given twenty unnumbered checks along with the list indicating to whom and for what amounts the checks are to be written. Patients should number the checks and fill out all of them. The signature should be included.

Now give each patient a check register. Have each person fill one out. When they are done, they should turn in the checks and the sheet indicating to whom the checks were written. They should keep the check register.

During the week, take a quick look at the checks to make sure that the basic procedure for filling them out was correct. Do not check for transposition errors, unsigned checks, or unnumbered checks. Leave these "real life" errors in the checks. Simply make sure that the basic procedure was followed correctly.

Tell the patients to bring the register in one week later. At that time, give them back their checks and a copy of the bank statement. Have them balance the checkbook.

Discussion

Did anyone lose the check register? How does this correlate with the way they handle their finances and other important matters in real life?

FIGURE 7.1.

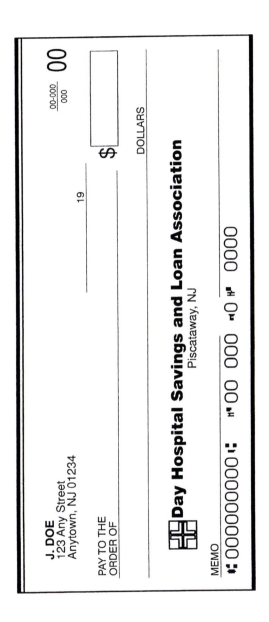

Where did they struggle in the process of balancing the checkbook? This is basically a didactic issue—just help them to learn.

Note: If you struggle with balancing your own checkbook, you might want to get that handled first before doing this with the patients.

TABLE 7.1. List of People to Whom Checks Are to Be Made

1. Deposit	$888.24	1/02/98
2. John Jones	$20.02	1/02/98
3. Grandma's Grocery	$49.48	1/02/98
4. Phone Co. of NJ	$55.55	1/06/98
5. Ernie's Electric Co.	$24.12	1/06/98
6. Crazy Credit Card Co.	$77.00	1/06/98
7. Day Hospital Savings and Loan	$134.90	1/06/98
8. Super-Crazy Credit Card Co.	$80.88	1/06/98
9. Mary Smith	$20.00	1/11/98
10. Void (check incorrectly made out, torn up, and thrown away)		
11. Gert's Gas	$18.18	1/12/98
12. Grandma's Grocery	$52.44	1/12/98
13. Cash	$30.00	1/13/98
14. Cash	$25.00	1/16/98
15. Grandma's Grocery	$8.09	1/17/98
16. Flo's Flowers	$23.00	1/20/98
17. Books on End	$26.99	1/20/98
18. Cash	$10.00	1/20/98
19. Vinnie the Vet	$88.88	1/25/98
20. Gert's Gas	$17.01	1/28/98
21. A Rose By Any Other Name	$28.77	1/29/98

Table 7.2

DAY HOSPITAL SAVINGS AND LOAN

Account Number 000111222	John/Jane Doe 123 Any Street Anytown, NJ 01234	Page 1
Office: Piscataway		Account Type: Regular
Phone: 123-456-7890		

Date		Checks and Other Debits		Deposits and Advances		Balance
1/02		20.02				36.04
1/02				888.24		924.28
1/02		49.48				874.80
1/06		55.55				819.25
1/06		24.12				795.13
1/06		77.00				718.13
1/06		134.90				583.23
1/06		80.88				502.35
1/11		20.00				482.35
1/12		18.18				464.17
1/12		52.44				411.73
1/13		30.00				381.73
1/16		25.00				356.73
1/17		8.09				348.64
1/20		23.00				325.64
1/20		26.99				298.65
1/20		10.00				288.65
1/25		88.88				199.77
1/28		17.01				182.76
1/29		28.77				153.99

Previous Statement Date	Taxpayer ID	Average Daily Collective Balance	Number Items Enclosed	Interest Earned This Year	Tax Withheld This Year	Period Ending Date
12/17/97	12345	$457.40	21	0	0	1/29/98
Previous Statement Balance	Total Checks/ Other Debts	Total Deposits and Other Credits	Service Charge	Interest Earned This Month	Tax Withheld This Month	Present Balance
$56.00	$790.31	$888.24	0	0	0	$153.99

Chapter 8

Social Skills

In this book I distinguish *social skills* from *socialization*. I define *social skills* as those skills necessary to be able to socialize effectively. These skills include assertiveness, anger management, teamwork, articulating an opinion, etc. Patients may *attempt* to socialize with others but, with poor skills, they will alienate others. Another possibility is that poor social skills will lead the patients to retreat from social situations that they find overwhelming. For example, if they have no idea how to behave at a wedding reception, they will not accept wedding invitations. If they lack skills in assertiveness, they will retreat when supervisors challenge them.

On the other hand, it is possible to know the proper way to manage social situations, but still shy away from them for any number of reasons (poor self-esteem, a need to hide major facts about their lives from others, etc.). People who know how to behave at wedding receptions may turn down wedding invitations anyway because they are shy. This chapter of the book is about social skills. Chapter 9 addresses the reluctance to socialize (socialization).

Soothing the Savage Beast is a group about anger, but it is not a traditional group about anger management. It is a group about managing one's own feelings in the face of being with another angry person. I designed this group after a room full of patients all indicated that they were terrified when someone close to them became angry with them. That is the beauty of program design. You can see what patients need and invent a group specifically to meet those needs.

Impromptu Speaking is a group designed to help patients with "social chit-chat." It is not a group for grossly psychotic people but definitely is not limited to the very high functioning either.

I held my breath the first couple of times I did Stating Your Case. People have concerns about discussing controversial issues in normal social gatherings, let alone in a day hospital with psychiatric patients. I found, however, that the group, because of its potential volatility, is very helpful in teaching people to control themselves. You need to judge who can learn from this group without losing control (or without losing control to a detrimental degree—it could be a useful learning experience if someone lost control in a way that was safe). For example, I ran a group in which there was a lesbian who had not revealed her lesbian identity to the group. One of the patients raised the question about admitting gays to the military and made an impassioned argument against it. During the discussion, the lesbian described how difficult it was for her to sit quietly through that. This led to a discussion about the need to endure these types of situations in real life.

The Party is fun and should be included on a day when there has been a lot of heavy-duty clinical work and the group needs something light.

Group Artistry is also intended to be light unless people are overly concerned about their lack of artistic ability. Conflict Resolution Skits are also fun provided you do not have a roomful of people with flat affect, which happened to me once. I handled the situation by becoming histrionic, which elicited a little bit of affect.

I designed What's Wrong with This Picture? to demonstrate that movie groups can be used for almost anything. In this group, movie clips are shown in which the characters demonstrate bad manners. The group is asked to discuss the problems they see with the characters' behavior.

SOOTHING THE SAVAGE BEAST

Introduction of Theme

Opening Questions

In this group we will explore the issue of anger. The focus, unlike most groups about anger, will not be about controlling our own anger. Instead we will look at our reactions to angry people.

How many of you are afraid of angry people? How do you react to the angry people in your lives?

Additional Comments

Often we approach the problem of dealing with angry people by trying to figure out ways to control them. It may be that we try to placate them or get away from them. We may make ourselves responsible for preventing their angry outbursts. These approaches are based in fear and usually do not work. These strategies magnify our fear of the explosive person who, we believe, has to be controlled. In this group, we will look at how to manage ourselves—not the angry person—in the face of the other's anger.

This is not to say that fear is never appropriate or that fleeing is never the right response. If someone is in a drunken rage and is about to hit you, you should be afraid and get out of the way. You may want to leave a relationship in which someone is always hitting you when drunk. The trick is to distinguish between genuine danger and fear that is out of proportion to the real danger.

Remember that we carry every relationship with us in our minds. Often we project our beliefs and feelings related to one relationship onto other people. For many who have lived with a chronically angry person, the old feelings associated with that person crop up again every time someone gets angry. One problem is that we may be adults experiencing anger through the eyes of a frightened child.

Introduction of Movie

We will use cuts from the Walt Disney version of *Beauty and the Beast* to help us in our discussion of anger. This movie is based on an old fairy tale. A prince who was mean and selfish once encountered an enchantress who, after being rebuffed by the prince, turned him into a beast. The spell could be broken only if he loved someone who loved him in return. If not, he would remain a beast forever.

The "Beauty," named Belle, meets the Beast while searching for her father who is imprisoned in the beast's castle for trespassing. Belle agrees to take her father's place and to live in the castle with the Beast forever. The story is about Belle's relationship with the Beast and what these two learn from each other.

Movie Cuts and Questions

BEAUTY AND THE BEAST

Cut 1

Belle's father was being chased by wolves. He saw the castle and took shelter there to get out of the cold and to be safe from the wolves. In this scene we will see what happens.

> Papa encounters Lumière (candlestick) and Cogsworth (clock). He sits in the Beast's chair and starts sipping tea when the Beast discovers him, intimidates him, and jails him. (Counter at approximately **17:11-20:25**.)

Questions

Does this beast remind you of anyone in your life? Who are the beasts in your life?

Take note of everyone's fear of the Beast and how they cope with him. How does Lumière cope with him? Cogsworth? And Papa? What kinds of reactions do you have to the beasts in your lives?

Additional Point

Let's take a closer look at the Beast and his reactions. First, note his paranoia. Belle's father came into the castle for safety. The Beast states, "So, you've come to stare at the Beast, have you?" He already has assigned a motive to the father's presence, one which conforms to his own poor self-esteem, shame, and self-loathing.

Question

Look at the beasts in your life. How do you think they feel about themselves?

Cut 2

Let's look at another facet of the Beast—his poor interpersonal skills. The Beast is so used to being a beast that he doesn't know how to be a gentleman.

> The father is allowed to go home and the Beast leads Belle to her room in the tower. He makes some clumsy attempts at compassion. He is first rather gruff with Belle about the room. Lumière is encouraging him to say something nice to her. He starts out all right but quickly loses his temper about the west wing. Lumière encourages him to ask Belle to dinner. Instead he says, "You will join me for dinner! That's not a request!" (Counter at approximately **22:50-29:28**.)

Questions

What do you think of the Beast? Why does he behave like this? Does this shed any light on the beasts in your lives?

Cut 3

Let's look at another kind of beast—the arrogant kind.

> Gaston arrogantly asks Belle to marry him. She turns him down, making him look like a fool in public. This only heightens his own insecurity. Then Gaston and the others sing a song about how macho Gaston is. (Counter at approximately **20:25-22:43**.)

Questions

Is Gaston self-confident? Is he insecure? How do you know? Does he resemble anyone you know?

Cut 4

> The Beast is pacing by the fireplace waiting for Belle to join him for dinner. He states, "She's so beautiful and I'm so—

well look at me!" Mrs. Potts states, "You must help her to see past all that." Beast responds, "I don't know how." (Counter at approximately **36:09-37:20**.)

Question

What do you notice about the Beast's self-esteem?

Cut 5

The Beast is being coached to be a gentleman. (Counter at approximately **37:20-35:50**.)

Question

Was this a success or a failure? Why?

Cut 6

Belle goes to the west wing. The Beast discovers her and loses his temper. She flees in terror, despair, and anger. (Counter at approximately **46:11-49:56**.)

Questions

When have you fled from an angry person? Was there something else you could have done?

Cut 7

In this interchange Belle stands her ground with the Beast. He responds openly and seems to hear her. Belle thanks the Beast for saving her life. (Counter at approximatley **52:11-53:07**.)

Questions

When have you behaved assertively with a beast? What happened? With what situations could you do that now? (You might wish to do some role-play here.)

What about looking for something good in the beast and complimenting him or her? Could you do this without expecting anything in return? After all, you may not get a positive response from someone with such poor self-esteem. Could you keep from personalizing a negative response?

Cut 8

In the following three scenes things improve between Belle and the Beast. When looking at these scenes see if you can figure out why.

> The Beast gives Belle a gift of a library. (Counter at approximately **54:48-56:49**.)

Discussion

Discuss the role giving plays in the Beast's healing. (He takes the attention off himself and puts it on someone else.)

Cut 9

> The Beast can't eat with a spoon. Belle accommodates him by drinking out of the cereal bowl. (Counter at approximately **56:49-57:29**.)

Discussion

Discuss the role of compassion and compromise in healing this relationship.

Cut 10

> Belle teaches the Beast to feed the birds. Belle and the Beast are falling in love. (Counter at approximately **57:29-59:24**.)

Questions

Why are things getting better between them? What might you learn from them?

Homework

Choose one beast in your life, past or present (preferably present). Write one paragraph describing the person's "beastliness."

Write another paragraph describing one or two good things about this person. Mention any efforts the person has made to learn to improve his or her skills. Even if this person was horrendous, try to think of one good thing that s/he did and write about that.

Think of a time in your life when you behaved like a beast. How were you feeling? How do you feel about it now? Can you forgive your own beastliness?

IMPROMPTU SPEAKING

Preparation

Have topics for discussion written on index cards. The topics should be broad enough to be usable by someone with a small fund of knowledge. Some suggested topics include television shows, books, something funny, anything in the news, pets, and music. Do not use controversial topics (e.g., religion or politics) or topics that require any complicated analysis (e.g., foreign affairs or economy).

Activity

Ask each patient to take a card and speak in front of the room on that topic for two minutes. Coach him or her as s/he speaks. Be on the lookout for the following: eye contact, fund of knowledge, volume of voice, posture, and ability to carry a conversation.

Remember to be extra supportive, as speaking in front of a group is frightening even for people who are not struggling with psychiatric problems.

STATING YOUR CASE

Preparation

You will need to make a copy of the Objectives/Discussion Questions sheet for each patient (see page 135). You will also need to have index cards with the issues printed on them (see pages 135-136).

Activity

Begin by going over the objectives on the "Objectives/Discussion Questions" sheet with the patients. Have some discussion about the objectives and make sure that they are thoroughly understood.

Give each patient an index card with an issue written on it. The patient is first to argue the question one way, and then to argue it the opposite way. This means that patients will be called upon to argue a point of view that they don't believe in. They are to do this seriously, considering compassionately what someone else might think. Everyone else is simply to listen as each patient speaks; there should be no cross-talk or arguing from others about the issues.

Patients should note their reactions as others speak.

EXAMPLE

Issue: Do you believe in the right to life or the right to choose?

Answer 1: I believe in the right to life because I believe that the fetus is a living being. That fetus doesn't have a say. If he or she did have a say, I believe the fetus would ask for his or her life.

Answer 2: The right to choose is a valid option because everyone has to decide this issue individually. It's possible to choose not to abort for a moral reason. If the government starts telling us how to make all of our moral choices, we are in trouble.

A person arguing these two cases would first argue the one he/she believes in and then argue the opposite.

Discussion

Use the discussion questions.

STATING YOUR CASE

Objectives

1. To listen to controversial issues without losing control of your emotions; to allow others to have their opinions.
2. To state your case clearly and convincingly.
3. To develop compassion for those with views different from your own.
4. To think critically about various issues.
5. To take risks.

Discussion Questions

1. Which issues upset you? Which ones brought up other feelings? How did you handle those feelings?
2. How do you handle your feelings about opinions of others in your life, such as your spouse, parents, employers, etc.?
3. How do you think you did in stating your case clearly? In what areas of your life do you have difficulty stating your case?
4. How do you rate yourself in the area of compassion?

Issues for Discussion

1. Do you believe in the right to life or the right to choose?
2. Should gays be allowed to serve in the military?
3. Should religion be allowed in public schools?
4. Should there be a cap on spending for political campaigns?
5. Should we have the death penalty?
6. Should refugees be allowed in the United States?
7. Should the U.S. intervene militarily in the problems of other countries?
8. Should money be spent to give therapy to sex offenders?
9. Do you believe in euthanasia?
10. Do you believe in monogamy or open relationships?
11. Should we limit the import and sales of foreign products?

12. Should cigarette smoking be banned in all buildings?
13. Argue in favor of a particular religion. Then argue against it. If you prefer you can use atheism or agnosticism.
14. Should we limit medical care and resources for those who are terminally ill?
15. Should we consider seriously the claims of alternative medicine?
16. Is affirmative action still valid?
17. Should we emphasize celibacy in teaching people about protecting themselves against AIDS and other sexually transmitted diseases?

THE PARTY

Preparation

The day room should be set up like a living room in which there will be a party. There should be appropriate (not too loud) music, coffee or tea, cold beverages, little treats, etc.—you decide. There should be chairs nicely arranged and plenty of room for people to mill around.

Tell patients the day before that you will be simulating a party. Ask them to dress the way they would dress for a party. They can even bring a food item or beverage if they wish. (Make sure they know it cannot be alcoholic.)

Activity

Patients are to mill around the room and socialize the way they would at a real party. Explain to them that you may intervene and coach them.

Instruct patients that they are not to discuss matters relating to their illness (e.g., hospitals, medications, therapists, etc.).

Notice the following:

- How the patients dressed
- Hygiene
- Who is withdrawing
- Appropriateness of conversation
- General etiquette, especially with food
- People who spend the entire time with one person

End the group with a discussion about the patients' social lives and how they might use what they learned in this simulation when they encounter real life situations.

GROUP ARTISTRY

Preparation

Hang up three pieces of very large paper, preferably white. Put out plenty of materials for artistry including magic markers, colored pencils, glitter, glue, etc.

Activity

Divide the group into three teams. Instruct the group to come up with one theme that can be expressed in three parts. Each of the teams will draw one part of the theme on one of the hanging papers. They will present their work to the group when finished.

Therapist's Observations

1. Did the entire group of patients decide on a theme or did they go off in three different directions without consulting one another? Did any of the groups forget that they were part of one large group?
2. Were there individuals who insisted on their own ideas, forgetting to include the group? For example, were there people who started drawing without consulting the group? Did they persist even when the group protested?
3. Were there individuals who took the bulk of the responsibility for the group? Who were the leaders? What was their leadership style?
4. Where there individuals who didn't participate? Did they know how to assert themselves in the group? Did they try to assert themselves and give up? Did the group notice this?
5. Were there individuals who shied away from the assignment because they were not artists? How much perfection did they demand of themselves? How did they feel about exposing their relative lack of artistic skill?
6. How did people treat the materials? Did anyone hog them? Did everyone remember to put them away? Were they neat? Did they work slowly and carefully or just slap something together?

7. What theme was chosen by the group as a whole? What sub-themes were chosen? Why did the group choose this theme?

Discussion

Lead a discussion about the group dynamics after each team has presented its picture.

CONFLICT RESOLUTION SKITS

Preparation

Three scenarios follow that could be used for conflict resolution. You will note that each scenario depicts the problem but not the solution. It is up to the patients to invent the solution. Of course, more than one solution can be invented!

You are welcome to use these scenarios; however, it would be better if you wrote some of your own that depict situations you think a specific group of patients has faced in the past or will face in the future. This will make the group far more meaningful. You might seek input from others on the staff, especially those who are working individually with the patients. The skits are very easy to write—you don't need to be Shakespeare to do it.

Activity

Have patients come to the center of the room and read the lines in one of the scenarios. Ask them to continue with the scenario from where the lines end. You can intervene whenever you feel it is appropriate. You can also start group discussion and have others step in to play one of the parts.

For extremely shy patients, I sometimes have one or two fellow patients stand next to them and coach them while the skit is in progress. We once had a very aggressive man who was playing the role of a merciless boss. The woman who was playing the employee was extremely withdrawn and helpless. I had three other patients stand around her and give her the lines. In this case it took four people to stand up to this particular boss! At first the patient was only saying what her coaches told her to say, but as the skit progressed, she became more bold and began adding lines of her own.

CONFLICT RESOLUTION SKIT

Scenario #1

Fran sits at her desk working hard. She is organizing papers and writing. After a moment or two, Bess walks into the room.

Bess: Hi, Fran. God, what a morning! I cannot believe I'm only a half hour late.

Fran: (Slightly annoyed) Hi, Bess.

Bess: Fran, the baby's sick again. I've got to take him to the doctor. The only appointment he had is for 3:00 today. Please be a dear and cover the meeting for me today.

Fran: Bess, I can't.

Bess: Fran, please! The baby's really sick. I've got to go.

Fran: This is the fourth time this month you asked—or insisted— that I cover for you. I've got work of my own to do.

Bess: Well, what can I do? I'd do the same for you if tables were turned.

Fran: Bess, I can't keep doing this. It's not fair.

Bess: I know it's been hard for you and I really am sorry. Look, let's not argue. We're a team, right?

* * *

Scenario #2

Merv comes home from the office to find his wife very depressed.

Merv: Hi, honey. (Walks into the kitchen, gets a drink, comes back into the living room) Aren't you cooking dinner?

Gert: (Shakes head no)

Merv: What's the matter now?

Gert: Just having a bad day. I have no energy.

Merv: Dammit, Gert, you do this all the time! Why can't you just pull yourself together?

Gert: I can't help it, Merv.

Merv: Yes you can! You're just not trying! Do I have to do everything around here?

Gert: You don't understand.

Merv: (Cutting her off) *You* don't understand. You've got to try harder!

*   *   *

Scenario #3

Blanche, Fred's mother, comes to visit Fred. She rings the bell. Fred opens the door.

Blanche: (Hugging him) Oh, hello dearest. What took you so long to answer the door?

Fred: Mom, I came right away to the door.

Blanche: Well, never mind. I'm just glad to see you. (Sits down) Honey, do you have some coffee?

Fred: (Annoyed) I was just making some, Mom.

Blanche: Why do you sound irritated?

Fred: (Softly) Never mind.

Blanche: What do you mean, never mind?

Fred: (Louder) Drop it, Mom, OK?!

(After some silence)

Blanche: Well, I came over to tell you about Christmas. We're going to gather around noon and dinner will be around 1:30.

Fred: Mom, I'm not sure about my Christmas plans yet.

Blanche: What do you mean? Aren't you going to be with the family? Of course you are.

Fred: I've had a couple of invitations.

Blanche: But *they're* not your family. And I know you love your family.

WHAT'S WRONG WITH THIS PICTURE?

Introduction of Theme

Today we will discuss social graces. What is meant by "social graces"? How can we learn them?

Introduction of Movies

We will use two movies to discuss this. The first is *Big*. In this movie, a little boy turns into a grown man. However, he is a little boy in a grown man's body. We will see how he behaves at a company party.

Forrest Gump, the second film, is about a man who is mentally challenged. We get to see the world from his point of view. In the scene that we will watch, he received honors from the president for his football playing. We'll see how he behaves at that party.

Movie Cuts and Questions

BIG

Cut 1

> The protagonist, Josh, arrives at a company party. He arrives inappropriately dressed. He licks the cheese out of the celery and dips his vegetable into the dip five or six times after biting each time. He eats a piece of baby corn (the kind in salads) as if it was regular corn on the cob, puts the "cob" in a napkin, and flings it to the side of the table. He and his friend try some caviar, which he hates. He spits it out on the floor, making all kinds of noise. He wipes his mouth out with a napkin and asks for a milkshake. (Counter at approximately **48:30-53:30**.)

Question

What problems in social grace did you notice in this clip?

FORREST GUMP

Cut 1

Forrest is at the presidential party for athletes voted to the all-American football team. He drinks sixteen Dr. Peppers very fast and then lets out a loud burp. Then he stands in line, wide-eyed, dancing around like he has to go to the bathroom. When the president asks him how he feels, he responds, "I've got to pee." (Counter at approximately **34:45-36:00**.)

Questions

What problems with social grace did you notice in this clip?

Now imagine that you are at a party and you eat something that you really hate. How would you handle the situation?

Suppose you had to go to the bathroom very badly at an awkward moment. What would you do?

What would you do in the following cases?

1. You go to a wedding. In the middle of the reception, you feel the strong urge to leave even though you are eating dinner with others.
2. You have to go to a job interview. How would you dress?
3. You decide to go to church or synagogue. What social graces would be important?
4. You go to a birthday party. What should you do?

Chapter 9

Socialization

This chapter addresses the internal barriers that impede socialization: the fear of intimacy. One might argue that this has no place in a short-term program as it is a long-term issue. It takes most people many years to develop a sense of comfort with genuine intimacy. It takes psychiatric patients even longer. What I focus on in this chapter, however, is isolation. Isolation exacerbates depression and should, therefore, be a target of treatment, even short-term treatment. I don't expect that people will have many relationships of great depth by the end of their stay in a short-term program. Still, they may resolve to make one or two friends, or they may pick up the telephone and call someone with whom they lost contact when they became symptomatic. Their relationships with family members may improve. These gains may contribute to prevent future hospitalizations.

Close Encounters discusses the tendency to isolate, a problem very common among psychiatric patients. Relationship and Risk addresses the question of intimacy. It considers the tremendous risk involved in reaching out to others. Blind Picture is a therapeutic game that requires trust. It also requires that one be "present"; one must listen actively and be aware of one's partner in order to succeed with the task involved. The Size of the World, a drawing exercise, attempts to depict the nature of the patients' social network. Since everyone can stand some improvement of their social network, it is easy to justify including just about anyone in this group.

The Wall was inspired by a story with the same name by Gloria Jay Evans. I find this a very powerful group, especially for people who are depressed and isolated. I remember one woman who expressed very little in most of the groups I ran. When I did The Wall, she sobbed after I read part of the story about the woman's isolation. She kept saying, "That is me." As she stood in front of her paper, marker in hand, she kept crying and saying, "I can't do it." With much gentle encouragement, she drew a picture of a woman behind a large fence. She then began to discuss her isolation. This incident, as well as many others, reminded me that the group activities are not just activities to encourage discussions. They also have the power to open up Pandora's boxes.

CLOSE ENCOUNTERS

Introduction of Theme

Opening Questions

In this group, we will look at the issue of intimacy. Usually when people talk about having an intimate relationship with someone, they are talking about sex. Today I am using the word "intimate" in a broader way. I am talking about the quality of our relationships with others.

What does intimacy mean to you?

Do you think that people have to know each other for a long time to be intimate?

Under what conditions do you think intimacy is possible?

Introduction of Movie

We will use cuts from the movie *Home Alone II: Lost in New York* for this group. This movie involves a little boy named Kevin McAllister whose family vacations in Florida. Kevin, however, accidentally gets on the wrong plane and ends up in New York City by himself. While he is in New York he encounters a woman in Central Park. We will look at their relationship.

Movie Cuts and Questions

Cut 1

On the surface, intimacy sounds like a great thing. But most of us are frightened of it. We, therefore, take pains to avoid it. Most of us, to one degree or another, feel unsafe in the world. We often learn to relate to people as if they were potential enemies.

> Kevin sees scary people in Central Park. (Counter at approximately **104:40-106:20**.)

Questions

Does the world ever look this way to you? If so, how would you recognize a friend in a world like this?

Cut 2

Kevin meets the homeless woman. The scene ends with them agreeing to have hot chocolate together. (Counter at approximately **106:20-109:54**.)

Questions

What allowed these two people to move from distrust to trust? What would allow you to move from distrust to trust?

Cut 3

"I'm like the birds I care for. People pass me in the street. They see me, but they try to ignore me."

" . . . Whenever the chance to be loved came along again, I ran away from it. I stopped trusting people."

"I'm just afraid if I do trust someone I'll get my heart broken again."

Kevin made an analogy to rollerblades. He was afraid to get them dirty or ruin them so he left them in the box. Then he outgrew them. He said that the same thing can happen with a person's heart.

"Your heart might still be broken but it isn't gone. If it was gone you wouldn't be this nice." (Counter at approximately **109:54-113:42**.)

Discussion

Use the above quotes from the scene to promote discussion about intimacy in the patients' lives.

Cut 4

"I have been working very hard at keeping people away, haven't I?" (Counter at approximately **113:42-115:53**.)

Question

How do you keep people away?

Homework

What price do you pay for keeping people away?

In what ways, if any, would you be willing to begin increasing the intimacy in your relationships with others?

RELATIONSHIP AND RISK

Introduction of Theme

Opening Questions

In Close Encounters we looked at the question of intimacy—what it is and how we avoid it. In this group we will look more closely into the courage it takes to be in a genuine relationship with another and the risks we must take to be fully with other people.

What risks do you run in getting close to someone? Is it better to run the risks or to protect yourself? Why?

Introduction of Movies

We will use cuts from *The Karate Kid, Shadowlands,* and *Ordinary People* for this group. *The Karate Kid* is about a boy named Daniel who is beaten up by other boys in school several times. He meets an older Japanese man who teaches him karate and prepares him to have a karate contest with the boy who threatens him the most. We will look at some aspects of the relationship between the boy and his teacher.

Shadowlands is the true story of the relationship between a famous writer named C.S. Lewis and a woman named Joy Gresham. We will look at the way C.S. Lewis changed over the course of this relationship.

Ordinary People is about a boy named Conrad and his parents. Conrad lost his brother in a boating accident. This was so devastating to him that he even attempted suicide. In this story, Conrad forges a relationship with a psychiatrist named Dr. Berger. We will look at this relationship.

Movie Cuts and Questions

KARATE KID

Cut 1

Daniel and his teacher have a little talk about the terms of their relationship. Daniel is told that he must do whatever the teacher tells him to do without question. (Counter at approximately **53:13-56:30**.)

Questions

What do you think of this arrangement? Is it unfair? Is it necessary? Would you agree to such an arrangement? Why or why not?

Cut 2

In this cut Daniel is required to sand the floor and then paint the house. He finishes with a confrontation with his teacher in which he accuses the teacher of using him to do his work without teaching him karate. His teacher shows him this is not true. (Counter at approximately **1:10:24-1:18:30.**)

Questions

Now what do you think of the previously discussed arrangement between Daniel and his teacher? Was it unreasonable?

How do you know when to trust someone who is asking for an unreasonable amount of trust? What is an unreasonable amount of trust for you?

ORDINARY PEOPLE

Cut 1

Let's look at a relationship that is closer to home for you—the relationship of a patient to a therapist or psychiatrist.

This is Conrad's first visit with his psychiatrist. It is awkward. (Counter at approximately **16:51-21:13.**)

Questions

How do you think Conrad felt? How do you feel when you have to start with a new therapist or psychiatrist?

What risks do you run in your relationship with your therapist or psychiatrist?

Cut 2

This is the scene where Conrad has his big breakthrough. (Counter at approximately **1:39:01-1:46:21.**)

Questions

What role did the psychiatrist play in making it possible for Conrad to experience this breakthrough? What role did Conrad's trust in the psychiatrist play?

How much risk will you take in the therapeutic relationship?

SHADOWLANDS

Cut 1

> In this scene, C.S. Lewis and Joy Gresham are married in a civil ceremony. There is no ring. The marriage is cold and formal. C.S. Lewis leaves quickly after the ceremony. (Counter at approximately **1:03:30-1:06:48**.)

Questions

How do you think these two felt? Why do you think the ceremony was so cold? What would he have had to risk to be warmer?

In what ways are you distant in your relationships? What would you have to risk to be warmer?

Cut 2

C.S. Lewis and Joy Gresham are married again in this scene, this time by a priest in the hospital where Joy is recovering from cancer. This ceremony is warm. (Counter at approximately **1:23:38-1:28:34**.)

Questions

What difference do you see between this scene and the last? What risks did they take? How do you think they will cope with the risks?

Homework

What risks, if any, are you willing to take in your relationships? How will you cope with the risks, especially with the disappointments?

BLIND PICTURE

Preparation

Attach very large pieces of drawing paper to the wall. Put out plenty of materials for drawing. Don't use anything that will permanently ruin clothes, the wall, or other materials in case there are any mishaps. Obtain blindfolds (large pieces of cloth will do if you don't have blindfolds).

Activity

Divide the patients into groups of four.

Blindfold one of the group members (a higher-functioning patient who is not paranoid). This person will draw a picture by listening to the verbal instructions given by the other three members. The instructors are not allowed to take the drawer's hand or help him or her draw at any point.

After the pictures are done, each group will present their picture and discuss the group process.

Discussion

Discuss trust issues.

How well did the blindfolded person listen? Did the blindfolded person draw what s/he was thinking about or what he was told to draw? How much interpretation was involved?

How well did the other team members communicate? How well did they work as a team?

THE SIZE OF THE WORLD

Preparation

Have plenty of drawing paper, markers, chalk, and other art materials on hand.

Activity

You can begin either with this story or any other story you know that illustrates a similar point. This is a true story from my childhood.

Story

Once my grandmother took my sisters and me for a walk. I was approximately five years old. At the time I thought there were about ten people in the whole world and that most of them lived in my house. While we were walking, I heard a total stranger call, "Lois! Lois!" I asked my grandmother why she was calling me. My grandmother explained that she was calling someone else. "But Lois is *my* name," I exclaimed. My grandmother explained that there were so many people in the world that names had to be used more than once. I was incensed. At the same time, I realized that there were really about one hundred people in the world, not ten.

Discussion

The world is quite large. Several billion people live in it. The size of *our* world, however—the one that each of us lives in—is much smaller. There are fewer people in it. There is less in it geographically. Because some people have traveled around the world, the geography of their world is large. Others may have never left their hometowns. The geography of their world is small. Some peoples' worlds include many experiences, others' very little.

Have the patients discuss this notion until you are satisfied that they understand it.

Activity

Instruct each patient to draw a picture of his or her world. They should begin by drawing a boundary. It could be a large circle, a square, the shape of a state or country—anything they like.

The patients should then draw on the inside of the boundary those people, things, and so on that are currently a part of their world. Right outside the boundary should be drawn those people, things, and so on, that are just out of reach—those things they desire but they can't quite attain. Far outside the boundary should be drawn those things that seem difficult to reach. (See Figure 9.1.)

For example, a person might draw pictures depicting her parents, with whom she lives, inside the boundary. She might draw a picture of a girlfriend or boyfriend just outside the boundary if she desires this type of relationship and believes she could achieve it in the near future. She might draw a picture of Japan far on the outside if she has relatives in Japan that she thinks about but believes she will never see.

Give patients plenty of time for this exercise. Be sure to stay in the room as they draw; don't leave and come back later. Some patients will struggle with the abstract aspects of this exercise and will need some extra instruction.

If some patients feel too self-conscious about drawing pictures, they can write words instead (e.g., write "mother" instead of drawing a picture).

Discussion

Have each patient present his or her picture. Note the following and make the appropriate interventions:

1. Is the inside of the boundary "people-less"? Is it "friend-less"? If so, how might more people or friends be added inside the boundary?
2. Are all the people in the boundary related to mental health institutions (doctors, nurses, day hospital staff, etc.)? If so, is there some way of including at least one person outside of this network?
3. If the person is recovering from addiction, is AA, NA, or a similar group depicted? Where is it?

FIGURE 9.1.

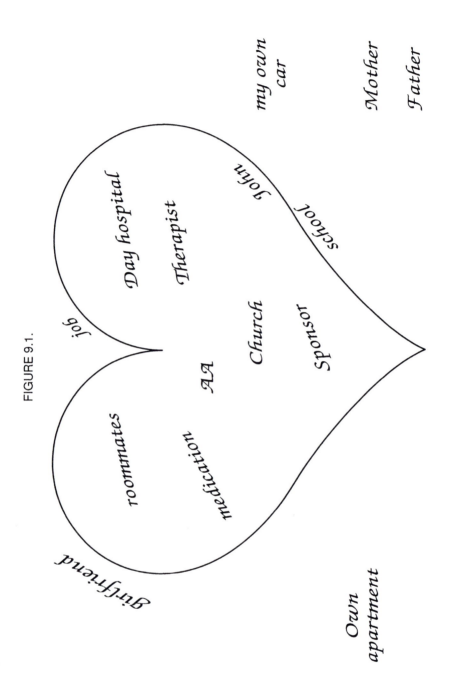

roommates

medication

AA

girlfriend

job

Day hospital

Therapist

Church

Sponsor

John

school

my own car

Mother

Father

Own apartment

4. Where is career or school in the picture?
5. Are any hobbies in the picture?
6. Is there a way of putting the things just outside the boundary inside the boundary?
7. Where is the family of origin in the picture?
8. Is anyone who is deceased in the picture? If so, where? How is the person's death being reconciled?
9. What role does romance play in the picture? Is this appropriate? Is it satisfying?
10. Is anything that you know to be an important part of the patient's life left out of the picture? If so, why?

THE WALL

Preparation

For this group, you will need to purchase the book titled *The Wall* by Gloria Jay Evans (Waco, Texas: Word Books, 1977). The book is religious in nature. You will obviously not be able to use the religious content in a secular program. The first half of the book, however, which has no religious content, is an excellent depiction of how someone builds an inner wall. You may, therefore, either use only the first half of the book or use the entire book as you wish.

You will also need to hang up one piece of large paper on the wall for every patient in attendance. Put out magic markers, colored pencils, and other art supplies.

Activity

Begin by explaining the theme of the group: isolation. Then read the first half of the book up to the part that states, "Your wall is ugly! It is twisted and misshapen!" Stop to get feedback from the group about how they relate to the protagonist.

In the next section of the group, have each patient draw a picture of his/her "wall." Explain that it does not have to be a literal wall, although it can be. They should draw pictures to illustrate whatever it is they use to separate themselves from others. They should be given plenty of time for this. Some groups require up to one-half hour; others are done in ten minutes.

Ask each person to present his/her picture to the group, explaining what s/he drew and why. Use clinical interventions at this point as you see fit.

Once all the pictures have been presented, have patients discuss how they might take down one tiny piece of the wall. Emphasize that you do not want them to tear the walls down. Their walls are their own and they may keep them up for as long as they are needed. You are, instead, looking for the key to removing one tiny stone.

If desired, this can be assigned as a homework question and discussed during homework review.

Note: Patients whose thinking is concrete may have difficulty with the assignment because it is abstract in nature. You can try to communicate the assignment in various ways. The following two examples have been useful to me under these circumstances:

> "Do you know what isolation is? Draw a picture that shows how you isolate yourself."

> "Do you shut other people out of your life? How? Draw a picture about that."

Something along these lines usually works. You may have to try a couple of times before you come across vocabulary that "hits."

Chapter 10

Self-Esteem

Self-esteem is an area often tackled in the day hospital milieu, sometimes by teaching techniques to increase self-esteem (such as affirmations) or by specific exercises designed to increase self-esteem (such as writing positive things about yourself). In this chapter, I include groups that allow people to explore their self-esteem. The groups afford clinicians a glimpse of patients' current self-image and offers a structure for change *without saying exactly what that change ought to be.*

As introduced in an earlier part of this book, movies allow patients to project their own concerns onto the characters. This allows them to talk about themselves without the threatening situation of having to see that they are talking about themselves. Sometimes I use interpretations or leading questions when I believe that the patient can benefit from it. Sometimes we just talk about the character and leave it at that.

Cinderella: Journey Toward Self-Esteem allows patients to explore the issue of emotional abuse and its relationship to self-esteem. Because this is such a loaded topic, it is helpful to have a set of characters onto whom patients can project their own concerns (Cinderella, wicked stepmother and stepsisters, rescuer prince).

Driving Miss Daisy: Accepting Support deals with the ambivalence of allowing ourselves to be supported and the ensuing loss of independence. Again, this is an extremely touchy issue. I have found it enormously helpful to use Miss Daisy as someone onto whom the conflict may be projected.

Rewriting Your Life allows people to present themselves in a fun fashion (as in a TV talk show). You will need to gauge the group, as some people simply find the video equipment too threatening. My experience has been that people initially find it threatening but loosen up after the first person does the mock interview. Lightening up yourself makes a huge difference in the mood of the group.

CINDERELLA: JOURNEY TOWARD SELF-ESTEEM

Introduction of Theme

Opening Question

In this group, we will examine our self-esteem. We won't just look at what level of self-esteem we have now. We will look at how a person might go from having little self-esteem to having a full appreciation of themselves.

What is self-esteem?

Introduction of Movie

For this discussion we will use the Walt Disney version of *Cinderella*. Some of you may not be familiar with Cinderella. Cinderella is a young woman who lives with her stepmother and two stepsisters, all of whom are rather mean. Cinderella is not mean. Her stepmother and stepsisters make a servant of her. The story tells how Cinderella gets out of this jam by meeting the prince, who falls in love with her and eventually marries her.

Movie Cuts and Questions

CINDERELLA

Cut 1

This beginning background about Cinderella reveals that she was "abused, humiliated" as well as being abandoned. She *was* "forced to become a servant in her own home." (Counter at approximatley **3:50-5:45**.)

Questions

Did you know this about Cinderella? Might this shed some new light on her behavior?

Cut 2

Take note of Cinderella's behavior in this scene.

> A mouse is found in a cup. The stepmother blames Cinderella and is verbally abusive, heaping a lot of work on her. Cinderella accepts this. (Counter at approximately **24:25-26:00**.)

Question

Is Cinderella kind, codependent, or both? Why?

Cut 3

This scene is presented as funny.

> The servant is abused by the king who seems to feel that he is entitled to be abusive because he is angry and frustrated. (Counter at approximately **26:00-28:30**.)

Questions

Do you think that the king was abusive? Why or why not?
What forms of abuse have occurred in your life?

Cut 4

> In this scene, Cinderella declares herself: "It says, 'Every eligible maiden.'" (Counter at approximately **30:50-32:35**.)

Questions

How do you suppose Cinderella felt when she did this? How would you have felt?

Cut 5

> There is more abuse and Cinderella hits bottom—she is in complete despair. It is then that the fairy godmother appears. (Counter at approximately **42:40-45:30**.)

Discussion

Discuss hitting bottom and what's possible from that.

Cut 6

The fairy godmother transforms Cinderella. (Counter at approximately **45:30-49:50**.)

Question

Imagine that you are Cinderella. You have just been transformed from a servant girl to a beautiful woman and you are going to meet the prince. How would you feel?

Cut 7

The fairy godmother declares the limit of this gift (midnight). Cinderella responds with gratitude: "It was more than I hoped for." (Counter at approximately **49:50-50:20**.)

Questions

Why do you think there's a limit on this gift? Could Cinderella handle it if there was no limit?

How much "goodness" could you handle?

Cut 8

Midnight comes and Cinderella is fleeing. As she does so, the coach turns into a pumpkin, the animals resume their original forms, and Cinderella is in servant's clothing again. She expresses gratitude for her experience, especially when she sees that she still has a glass slipper. (Counter at approximately **56:40-59:12**.)

Discussion

Is there a relationship between gratitude and self-esteem? If so, what do you think it might be?

Cut 9

Cinderella responds differently to her stepsisters, daydreaming and leaving the laundry in their hands. She walks off humming. (Counter at approximately **1:03:20-1:05:20**.)

Question

Why do you think Cinderella is responding differently to her family now?

Cut 10

There is one more act of cruelty: the stepmother trips the man who is holding the glass slipper. The man falls and the slipper breaks. Cinderella produces the other one. (Counter at approximately **1:14:15-1:15:34**.)

Questions

How would you describe Cinderella now?
What role did *she* play in getting to the point where she could become a princess?

Homework

Where do you see yourself in your journey toward self-esteem?
Describe your "royal self."

DRIVING MISS DAISY: ACCEPTING SUPPORT

Introduction of Theme

Opening Questions

This is a group about accepting support from others.

How do you feel about accepting others' support? What kinds of support are you willing to accept? What kinds are you unwilling to accept?

Introduction of Movie

We will use cuts from the movie *Driving Miss Daisy* to discuss this issue. Miss Daisy is a woman in her seventies who has been independent all her life. She has a strong personality. After she has an accident with her car, her son determines that she can't drive any longer and hires a driver named Hoke. The movie is about the relationship between Miss Daisy and Hoke.

Movie Cuts and Questions

DRIVING MISS DAISY

Cut 1

Miss Daisy refuses to meet Hoke. She has an argument with her son about it. (Counter at approximately **13:30-16:15**.)

Questions

What do you think of Miss Daisy's attitude? How do you think she feels?

Cut 2

This is a series of events with Hoke in which Hoke can do nothing right. He can't win with Miss Daisy. (Counter at approximately **16:15-24:50**.)

Questions

What do you think of Miss Daisy here? Why is she behaving like this?

Is there someone in your life with whom you can't win? Is there someone who can't win with you? If so, why?

Cut 3

Hoke reveals to Miss Daisy that he can't read. Miss Daisy teaches him to read the word "Bauer" on the tombstone. (Counter at approximately **35:30-41:41**.)

Questions

How do you think this seventy-year-old man felt about not being able to read? What do you think allowed Miss Daisy to interact better with Hoke? What did each have to give to the interaction to make it work?

Cut 4

This is the final scene in which Hoke feeds Miss Daisy her pie in the nursing home. It speaks for itself. (Counter at approximately **1:34:00-1:36:33**.) (end of film)

Discussion

Elicit reactions to the above.

Homework

What is the difference between support and codependence? Independence and stubbornness?

In what ways will you allow others to support you?

REWRITING YOUR LIFE

Preparation

For this group you will need audio-visual equipment. Test it in advance to make sure it works and to make sure that you know how to work it. You will also need about four toy telephones.

Be sure to have written permission from the patients to videotape even if you intend to destroy the tape right after the group.

Activity

This group is a simulation of a talk show with the patient as the "guest" and the therapist as the "host." The following is an outline for a script which might be useful.

- "Good afternoon and welcome to another addition of 'Central New Jersey.' Our guest for today is _____. _____, welcome to the show."
- "Give the viewers an overview of your life."
- "What common misperceptions do viewers have about you?" "What would you like the viewers to know about you?"
- "Talk about the future."
- "Tell us more about _____."
- "With what message would you like to leave the viewers?"

Have viewers call in using the toy telephones.

Discussion

While doing the interviews be aware of the following:

1. In what light did the patients present themselves?
2. Was there too much focus on mental illness?
3. What concerns did they project onto the "viewers"?
4. Was there a future orientation? What did the patients see for themselves in the future?
5. What role did others play in the description of their lives?

6. How conversant were they? How was eye contact? Volume?

7. What does the presentation say about their self-esteem?

Have the patients look at these questions and comment. You can coach the patients during the interviews or after. You can have patients repeat interviews after the coaching.

Homework

Imagine that you really are a guest on a TV show. Imagine the whole thing, seeing yourself in a positive light. This shouldn't be grossly unrealistic, but it should portray a picture of the present and future *you* that is admirable. Share this new *you* at the homework review.

Note: This homework should not be given to people who are actively psychotic or are struggling with grandiose delusions.

Chapter 11

Motivation

I don't know how many people consistently use motivational material in their day hospital programming. All material, if well used, is motivational. In this chapter, I introduce material that is specifically designed to instill patients with a sense of possibility about their lives.

A growing sense of despair often accompanies the management of a mental illness. In some cases, when the first break occurs, people still have a sense of hope about their future. As a matter of fact, I often need to slow these people down because they are all too eager to jump right back into their old activities, possibly endangering their stability. On the other hand, once people have been ill for many years—once they have lost a number of jobs or failed to get married and passed the age where they can have the children they wanted—there is often the sense that nothing is possible anymore, that one is doomed to the life of a "typical mental patient," which will involve nothing more than medication, side effects, sleep, and multiple hospitalizations.

I find myself wondering what role this despair plays in impeding recovery (or at least in limiting possibility in the people's lives). After all, people who are sure that they "can't do it" probably won't even try. Often, people who live with the constant thought that "I am a failure" won't try to succeed. It is with these thoughts in mind that I created the motivational series. What inspired me most about day hospital treatment was not the possibility of teaching people how to do their laundry or successfully reinforcing the need to take medication consistently, important though these may be. What inspired me was the opportunity to instill in the patients a sense of possibility about their lives.

It is important, as always, for one to be realistic. It is not my goal to set people up for failure with goals that are out of reach. Patients who are grossly psychotic are not encouraged to get their own apartment and a job. They might be encouraged, however, to try getting out of bed on their own in the morning.

New medicines create possibilities that did not exist in the past. I will never forget a patient who, after years of having a treatment-resistant psychosis, tried clozapine successfully. It was the first time in twenty years that he was not grossly delusional. His reaction? He was frightened out of his wits. He had no idea how to live without delusions. He had no idea who he was. He was frightened of responsibility, something that might be expected of him now that he was better. Part of him wanted to be well. Part of him wanted his old delusional system back.

The first group, Beyond Survival: Creating a Life Worth Living, addresses the issue of patients' ambivalence about being well. Running this group requires a great deal of clinical skill because patients may misinterpret the material. Guilt-ridden patients may use the material to augment their own sense of guilt about being psychiatrically ill. Or people may use the material to infer that "I can do anything" (even grossly unrealistic things). One must keep in mind that Colin, the protagonist, was perfectly able to walk; there was nothing wrong with him. One might discuss how he would have handled it if there had indeed been something wrong with his legs or back.

The Perils of Oz was created for a group of patients who erroneously believed that because they were in treatment they should feel better. Many of them noted that they felt worse, especially those who were dually diagnosed and had very little sobriety. The message of this group is, "Things may get worse. Don't quit!"

Portraits of Courage was designed to address the problem of people getting too comfortable in the day hospital and using it as an escape from the demands of life in the community. I'm Looking for Yoda was designed to help people view the idea of learning in a new light. It also addresses the issue of failure as a natural part of learning. The Captain of the Ship illustrates the point that we are in charge of our own experiences. Until people can begin to see that their experience of life comes from themselves rather than from outside forces, there is little hope for therapeutic change.

Against All Odds addresses the issue of fighting for something that seems impossible. The movie clips, based on two true stories, highlight the courage of people who weren't "supposed" to succeed.

The last two groups in this section, Gratitude: The Healing Ground and Awakening to Joy, were designed for the holiday season (Thanksgiving and Christmas respectively). Holidays are difficult for patients. Helping them to create a meaningful way to celebrate the holiday is important. Making the interventions therapeutic gives clients more than they would get from receiving only a gift or a turkey dinner at the hospital cafeteria. It helps to make the holiday authentic for them.

I have not been afraid to address existential issues with psychiatric patients. People sometimes believe that psychiatric patients have not developed enough emotionally to deal with such issues. I disagree. These issues are sometimes pressing for them. As a matter of fact, the question, "What is the meaning of my life?" or "What is my life for?" or "Why am I here?" is particularly salient for someone who missed many developmental milestones and knows that s/he will not be able to make the ordinary contributions to society. I personally know of one woman who recently killed herself. Shortly before that, she had been openly discussing the fact that she had not achieved what she wanted to in her life: marriage, children, job. She saw no meaning in her life. Unfortunately, she could not create a meaning that made her want to live. We cannot ignore this important issue when we work with psychiatric patients.

BEYOND SURVIVAL: CREATING A LIFE WORTH LIVING

Introduction of Theme

Opening Discussion

This group will examine our relationship with illness. Most people who are ill want very much to be well. Sometimes, however, there is a part of them that doesn't want to be well or, more correctly, that is afraid to get well. That may sound like a strange thing to say, but that is what we will examine today.

We will also look at the ways we are sometimes tempted to manipulate our illness when dealing with others.

Opening Questions

What do you think of what was said in our opening discussion? Do you think there are times when people use illness to manipulate others? How?

Note: You may think the discussion and questions too straightforward; however, my experience has been that people smile and nod their heads when this aspect of illness is discussed.

Introduction of Movie

The movie we will use for our discussion is *The Secret Garden.* This movie is about the relationship between a boy named Colin Craven and a girl named Mary Lennox. Mary Lennox was born in India but unfortunately lost both her parents in an earthquake. She came to England to be cared for by her uncle, Lord Craven. She heard wailing noises in the mansion but was told that these noises were the wind, a ghost, etc. She was far too smart for this and realized that she would have to do some detective work to find the source of the noise.

Movie Cuts and Questions

THE SECRET GARDEN

Cut 1

Mary finds the source of the noise, a wailing boy named Colin who of his own volition is shut away in a corner of the house. The two have a stormy meeting in which Mary confronts him about his manipulations. Among other things, Colin declares that no one can make him do anything because he is sick. (Counter at approximately **50:30-53:00**.)

Questions

What do you think of Colin?
Do you ever hold your illness over people's heads? If so, how?

Cut 2

Colin: "Everyone has to do as I say because I'm going to die."
Mary: "People who talk about dying are boring."
(Counter at approximately **52:32-53:00**.)

Questions

What do you think of Mary's comeback? What do you think of what Colin said?
What do you think about people who talk about suicide constantly? Why do you think they do it?

Cut 3

Colin is giving orders to staff. The manipulation is obvious.
Mary: "You're the one who's selfish. All you think about is yourself and feeling sorry for yourself."
Colin: "You'd feel sorry for yourself too if you had a lump on your back and you were going to die."

Mary: "You say things like that because you want people to feel sorry for you."
(Counter at approximately **1:02:00-1:03:10**.)

Questions

Do you ever want people to feel sorry for you? If so, why?

Cut 4

Colin screams. Everyone is powerless except Mary. She lays down the law. She also informs Colin that he has no lump on his back. (Counter at approximately **1:03:10-1:05:30**.)

Discussion

Note Colin's reaction when his assumption about dying is questioned by Mary.

Note: You may wish to replay this section. Colin feels threatened by the first response and nervously asks the nurse to confirm his view of his illness.

Question

What do you think of Mary here? Is she being mean? Why or why not?

Cut 5

Colin agrees to meet Dickon. Dickon comes in with animals. Then Colin goes outside for the first time. He decides that the garden will make him well. (Counter **1:07:25-1:11:41**.)

Questions

Do you see how Colin progressed from total isolation to moving out into the world? How might you do that?

Cut 6

Colin plants his first rose. He learns to walk and fails once. (Counter at approximately **1:15:31-1:20:37**.)

Question

Are you willing to fail as you learn something new?

Cut 7

Mary compares their thinking to thistles and roses. In the next scene, Colin walks. (Counter at approximately **1:23:30-1:24:39**.)

Homework

What are the thistles (negative thoughts) that keep you isolated? What roses (positive thoughts) could you add to your life now?

Examine your life very honestly. Do you sometimes use your illness to manipulate others? If so, how? Are you willing to change this?

THE PERILS OF OZ

Introduction of Theme

Opening Discussion

We often think that, as our treatment progresses, our lives will get easier. Problems will slip away. This is not always the case. We may think of ourselves as failures if things do not get better or if things get worse. Following are some examples of this phenomenon.

- A patient who stops drinking starts to experience intense anxiety at having to solve problems for the first time rather than drowning them with alcohol.
- A patient on clozapine once said, "When I was delusional, the bums in the street didn't bother me because I didn't notice them. Now they really upset me."
- A patient begins a job. She holds the job for three months and winds up back in the hospital. She feels like a failure even though she never held a job before.

Introduction of Movie

We will use the movie *The Wizard of Oz* to discuss this further. The movie is about a girl named Dorothy and her three friends, the Lion, the Scarecrow, and the Tin Man. All four of them are on a journey to Oz to ask the Wizard of Oz to grant them certain favors. Dorothy plans to ask the Wizard to send her home to Kansas (Dorothy is lost in Oz and doesn't know how to get back home). The Lion is cowardly and plans to ask for courage, while the Scarecrow plans to ask for a brain. The Tin Man will ask for a heart. We will enter the scene three-quarters of the way through the movie after they have journeyed a long way and survived many perils. They are almost at the Wizard's castle.

Movie Cuts and Questions

THE WIZARD OF OZ

Cut 1

The lion sings about what he would do if he was king of the forest. He is happy and full of energy. Right after that the entire group is in despair because the Wizard has refused them entrance. It appears that the entire journey was for naught. (Counter at approximately **103:56-108:30**.)

Question

When have you felt that you "traveled a long way" for nothing?

Cut 2

The group is walking through a scary hall to see the wizard. The Lion wants to turn back. They reach the Wizard and speak with him. The Wizard frightens them. He then tells them to bring him the broom of the wicked witch. (Counter at approximately **108:30-1:13:26**.)

Questions

Notice how things went from bad to worse, and that what appeared to be the end of a long journey was not.

When have your hopes been dashed in this manner? When have you been asked to do the "impossible," especially by someone in authority?

Cut 3

Dorothy and her friends are out in the woods. They encounter the sign saying "I'd turn back if I were you." The Lion tries to turn back but the others stop him. The witch sends her monkeys out to get them and they are carried off to the witch. (Counter at approximately **1:13:26-1:16:57**.)

Question

Suppose they decided to quit because things were supposed to get better for them after they got to Oz?

Cut 4

The witch decides to kill Dorothy. She turns the hourglass over and leaves Dorothy to die. (Counter at approximately **1:16:57-1:20:05**.)

Question

How are they doing now? (This should get a laugh.)

Cut 5

They face the witch. The Scarecrow gets stuffed again and sets off to find Dorothy. Toto runs away and comes back for the others. They try to escape with Dorothy. (Counter at approximately **1:20:05-1:25:05**.)

Question

When have you had to keep going even though it seemed impossible or ridiculous to do so?

Note: I would finish the group here. To show the film to the end brings a fairy tale feeling to it that takes away from the demonstration of difficulty. You don't want the patients saying, "Well we knew it would turn out fine in the end." If they do, ask, "Suppose the movie ended here (any of the difficult points)? Suppose it ended because they quit right here?"

Homework

Discuss a time when you quit because things got very hard. What might have been possible if you kept going?

Discuss a time when you kept going when things were hard. What would have happened if you quit?

PORTRAITS OF COURAGE

Introduction of Theme

Opening Question

What do you think courage is? Don't try to give a dictionary definition, but instead, speak about what it means to you personally.

Introduction of Movie

We will look at a couple of cuts from *The Sound of Music*. This movie is based on a true story. Maria starts out as a nun. Her superior realizes that she is not cut out for religious life and sends her to be a governess for a family in the area. The Captain is a widower with seven children. A string of governesses have all left quickly due to the Captain's strict, cold personality and the mischievous natures of the children. The movie is about the relationship between Maria, the Captain, and the children.

Movie Cuts and Questions

THE SOUND OF MUSIC

Cut 1

Maria stands up to the Captain. The children sing for the first time in a long time and the Captain joins them. He apologizes to Maria and asks her to stay after having fired her. (Reel 1, Counter at approximately **1:15:38-1:23:45**.)

Questions

What elements of courage do you see here?
Note: Make sure they pick up on Maria's assertiveness even in the face of risking her job, the children's singing, the Captain's singing, the Captain's hugging his children, and the Captain's courage to apologize.

Can you identify with any of these characters? How?

Cut 2

> Maria tries to go back to the abbey to run away from her fear about being in love with the Captain. The Mother Superior will not allow her to do this.
> Mother Superior: "These walls were not built to shut out problems." (Reel 2, Counter at approximately **22:52-25:50**.)

Discussion

This is a temporary lapse in courage. Note the role that support plays in success here. Maria is pushed to address her fear.

Questions

What happens when you try to push a challenge under the rug? Who in your life will push you to face your fears?

The day hospital walls were also not built to shut out problems. How have you been using the day hospital, the inpatient unit, or both to shut out problems?

Homework

What risks are you going to take *outside* of the day hospital while you are still in the day hospital program? When? Who will support you?

I'M LOOKING FOR YODA

Introduction of Theme

Opening Question

Today we will explore the issue of learning. Why do you think we would look at that issue in a day hospital? After all, this isn't a school.

Additional Comments

Our definition of learning is often constricted by our experience in public (or private) school. We think of learning as occurring in a classroom with a formal teacher. Outside of that situation, learning does not occur—or so we think.

How did you learn how to behave at the dinner table? Probably from your family. They gave you open messages ("don't play with your food") and informal messages (what you learned from watching others at the table).

How did you learn how to handle conflict? Probably in a very subtle manner—by watching others or observing the "family rules." For example, if you saw your mother give in to your father all the time, you learned that this is how a woman handles conflict with a man.

Actually we are always learning at every moment. We learn by interacting with others and experiencing the consequences of our interactions. We learn by observing others. We learn by reading the newspaper, and in many other ways.

Introduction of Movie

The Empire Strikes Back is the second in the Star Wars series popularized in the 1970s. Luke Skywalker, the protagonist, is a hero who has the ability to be a Jedi warrior in this science fiction movie. He has to learn, however, from a great Jedi master named Yoda.

Movie Cuts and Questions

THE EMPIRE STRIKES BACK

Cut 1

Note: Play these scenes one right after the other.

> Luke Skywalker first meets Yoda in this scene. Luke does not recognize his teacher because he thinks the teacher should look a certain way—like a great warrior. He thinks that Yoda is just a pain in the neck who is eating all of his food. (Counter at approximately **51:23-55:27** and **59:11-1:02:30**.)

Questions

What teachers in your lives have you failed to recognize?

We often acknowledge the opportunity to learn something in the day hospital. What opportunities for learning exist for you *outside* of the day hospital?

Cut 2

It isn't possible to face an entirely new situation outside the bounds of our normal comfort zone without being afraid. Unfortunately, this often leads us instinctively to avoid the things we fear.

> At one point Luke protests, "I'm not afraid." Yoda states, "You will be. You will be." (Counter at approximately **1:02:01-1:02:30**.)

Questions

What is the role of fear in learning?

What is at the edge of your comfort zone (what new situation do you fear, e.g., going to work)? How do you manage this fear?

Give examples of times when you were afraid to do something but you did it anyway.

How many of you are afraid of failure?

Cut 3

Failure is an inevitable part of learning. This is because you are trying something new, something at which you are not practiced.

When a baby first tries to walk, doesn't s/he fall many times? When a child first learns to ride a bike, doesn't s/he fall many times? Does this say something terrible about the baby or the child? Of course not. It is saying something positive—that the baby or the child is being courageous enough to break through to a new level of competence. This is true for adults as well. The first time you try your hand at baseball you strike out. You strike out many times. The point is to keep trying until you get it right. Let's see, for example, how our friend Luke Skywalker learns.

> While hanging upside down, he fails to pick up a stone by using his power. (Counter at approximately **1:13:00-1:13:47**.)

Cut 4

Despair is also a natural part of learning. Let's see how our friend Luke Skywalker fares.

> His ship is in the water. He exclaims, "Now we'll never get it out." Yoda states, "So certain are you? Always with you it can't be done." (Counter at approximately **1:13:47-1:14:02**.)

Question

What have you decided can't be done in your life?

Cut 5

> "All right. I'll give it a try."
> "No. Try not. Do. Or do not. There is no trying." (Counter at approximately **1:14:02-1:14:31**.)

Questions

What have you been "trying" to do without actually doing it? Discuss the futility of trying, considering, thinking about, etc.

Cut 6

As mentioned before, despair is a natural part of learning. The point is that, for Luke, despair is not the end, it is just momentary.

> Luke tries to raise the ship and fails. He goes off to a corner in total despair. (Counter at approximately **1:14:31-1:16:33**.)

Questions

What life challenges bring out despair in you?

Where did you give up in the past? Are you ready to forgive yourself and get up to bat again?

Cut 7

> "I don't believe it."
> "That is why you fail." (Counter at approximately **1:16:33-1:18:12**.)

Questions

What role does belief play in learning? Where is your disbelief? Are you willing to believe that you can learn to handle life's challenges?

Homework

Identify one *small* area in your life where you have refused to learn—where you keep "trying" without "doing."

Get up to bat! Take this item and do it. Write a paragraph about your experience afterward. If you fail, that is fine. Make that part of your paragraph.

AGAINST ALL ODDS

Introduction of Theme

This group will examine our relationship with hardship and calamity.

Have you ever noticed that you can take two people suffering from the same hardship, put them side by side, and discover that they will handle it very differently? Let's take cancer as an example. Two people can have the same medical diagnosis of cancer. One will fight ferociously to recover. Another will give up and die relatively quickly. On occasion, people who are "supposed to die" don't as a result of their fierce tenacity.

Opening Questions

What distinguishes the fighter from the one who gives up? Why would someone fight to live? Why would someone give up? Which person do you think you are?

Introduction of Movies

We will use cuts from two movies. The first is *My Left Foot.* This movie is based on the true story of a man named Christie Brown who was crippled. He was very poor. When he was young, there was thought to be no real hope for "cripples." He couldn't talk and couldn't move most of his body. We will see two clips demonstrating his tenacious spirit.

The other movie is *Rudy,* also based on a true story. This movie is about a man named Rudy Rudiger whose dream was to play football for Notre Dame. Since he was not very brilliant and had poor grades, this was not a likely possibility. Furthermore, he was small and didn't have great skills as a football player. He was so committed to his goal, however, that he achieved it against all odds.

Movie Cuts and Questions

MY LEFT FOOT

Cut 1

> In this cut, Christie attempts to write "1/16" on the floor with a piece of chalk. He fails to do so. His family fails to understand what he is trying to do. (Counter at approximately **17:02-19:00**.)

Question

Comment on Christie's attitude. How do you think he felt when he failed?

How do you feel when you fail? Does it make you want to give up? Give examples.

Cut 2

> Christie attempts to write "Mother" on the floor and succeeds. His family is elated and his father takes him to the bar. (Counter at approximately **25:13-29:11**.)

Questions

Why do you think Christie kept trying? What would keep you going in spite of failures?

Can you see a bit of yourself in Christie?

Movie Cuts and Questions

RUDY

Cut 1

> Rudy arrives on the football field at Notre Dame. He tells the workman that he will play on that field one day. He then

practically barges into the coach's office and informs him that he will play for Notre Dame the next year. He speaks as if it is a fait accompli. (Counter at approximately **32:12-36:05**.)

Question

What do you notice about Rudy's attitude? Do you think it is ridiculous to speak as if something is definitely going to happen even though it may not happen? Why would he speak that way?

If you were going to come into my office and tell me in no uncertain terms what you are going to accomplish next year, what would you say? Say it now.

Homework

Write your response to the question about what you are going to accomlish next year. Read it to yourself, out loud, at least once every day this week.

THE CAPTAIN OF THE SHIP

Preparation

This group does not require props. Following are five scenarios. Have the patients discuss each of them. Where appropriate, discussion questions follow.

Scenario #1

You are the captain of a ship. You are at sea. The wind kicks up and waves begin to swell. They get higher and higher. It starts to rain. What do you do?

Of course you sit back helplessly and hope that the ship doesn't sink. What else can you do? After all, is it your fault that there was a storm at sea while you were sailing? You're not in control of the weather, are you?

Scenario #2

You are driving along the highway and a drunk driver starts to drive the wrong way in your lane. What do you do? Do you sit back and accept your fate? Or do you swerve, driving wherever you must in order to avoid a crash? Do you sit back, taking your hands off the wheel, and say to yourself, "This is unfair. I shouldn't have to drive on a road with a drunk driver. I'm not going to do any more driving until he leaves"?

Scenario #3

You are in a car accident (maybe you couldn't avoid the aforementioned drunk driver). You are paralyzed from the waist down. What do you do with your life? Do you sit at home waiting for others to take care of you because, after all, it wasn't your fault that there was a drunk driver on the road? Isn't it unfair that you can't walk while others can? Doesn't that entitle you to relax and let others control your life?

Scenario #4

You grew up with abuse. Your childhood was traumatic. You never learned to feel good about yourself, you got poor grades in school, and barely got your high school diploma. You have few friends. Do you sit back and blame your parents? There is plenty of literature to support your position if you do. If your parents are responsible for your plight, what is your responsibility now?

Scenario #5

You are mentally ill. You have mood swings that are sometimes well controlled by your medication and sometimes not. You haven't worked in a number of years. You lost your last job in the middle of a manic episode. Currently you're depressed. You find it hard to get out of bed in the morning and it takes a great deal of energy for you to clean the house or cook your meals. You lost a lot of friends when you became ill—they just got tired of dealing with your depression.

Who or what is to blame for this? What is your responsibility for getting well? What is someone else's responsibility for your getting well? Whose? Who is responsible for managing your life? What does that mean in the face of circumstances you can't control? What about the fact that it is unfair?

Homework

Write two short stories. One will be the story of a person with your mental illness who doesn't take responsibility for managing his or her life. What does this person think? How does s/he behave? The other will be a short story of this same person, except that in this story s/he takes responsibility for managing his or her life.

If you prefer, the group can be divided into smaller groups to perform skits, written by them, in which they demonstrate the two situations mentioned above.

GRATITUDE: THE HEALING GROUND

Exercises in Thanksgiving

Preparation

For this group you will need a copy of Og Mandino's *The God Memorandum.* This may seem like an odd selection for a day hospital group, but the part that we will use is a portion of the "God Memorandum" in the back of the book.

Questions for Discussion

What do you think Thanksgiving is? What role do you think gratitude plays in your healing?

Let's look at the body, for example. How many of you take your body for granted? How many of you believe that your body basically doesn't work well for you?

Activity 1

Read the portion of *The God Memorandum* in the back of the book that pertains to the body. It mentions, for example, that you have 100 million receptors in your eyes as well as 24,000 fibers in each ear. Stop after each item for reactions and comments.

Have a discussion about the miraculousness of the human body.

Questions

How do you feel now about your body? What else might you be taking for granted?

Activity 2

Have patients go for a short, silent walk. They should look around them and make a mental note of what they perceive as beautiful. If they have problems with memory, they can take their notebooks and jot these things down. Emphasize that there is to be no talking and that the exercise is to be done seriously. Make sure that the walk is relatively short. Also emphasize that the group will be walking slowly to give people time to notice what is around them.

When you return have patients share what they noticed.

Question

For what new thing will you be grateful today?

AWAKENING TO JOY

Introduction of Theme

Opening Questions

Today we will be discussing joy. We will examine what inhibits joy and what promotes joy in life.

This is a time of year in which tradition holds that everyone is supposed to be joyful. Are you joyful? Why or why not? What is joy?

Introduction of Movies

We will use cuts from two movies. Most of the cuts will come from the 1988 version of *A Christmas Carol.*

A Christmas Carol is a famous story written by Charles Dickens. It is the story of a man named Ebenezer Scrooge who was very mean-spirited. He hated Christmas and just about everything else. He is visited Christmas Eve night by three spirits who, in a way, practice psychotherapy on him. These spirits attempt to help Scrooge become happy again.

The other movie we will look at briefly is *It's a Wonderful Life.* This movie is about a man named George Bailey who, at a time of despair, considers suicide. An angel saves him by showing him what life would be like in his town if he had never been born. He gets to see how many lives he has affected in a positive way by seeing what would and would not have happened if he weren't around.

Movie Cuts and Questions

A CHRISTMAS CAROL

Cut 1

In this cut we get to see Scrooge being nasty. He declares that Christmas is a "humbug," harasses someone who owes him money, and shoos away poor children. (Counter at approximately **0:11-5:20.**)

Questions

Do you see any of Scrooge in yourself? What do you think Scrooge is feeling?

Cut 2

Scrooge is with the Ghost of Christmas Past. He sees himself as a boy in school who was shunned by his father for many years. His sister comes to bring him home. He declares that his sister is the only one who loves him. He reveals that his mother has died.

"Nobody else ever cared for me. Nobody else ever will."
(Counter at approximately **23:00-26:10**.)

Questions

Does this give you some hint about what's hurting Scrooge? What's hurting you?

What do you notice about Scrooge's quote? (Point out the fatalistic thinking.)

Cut 3

Scrooge and Marley meet each other.

"I think the world is becoming a very hard and cruel place, Mr. Marley. One must steel one's self to survive it, not be crushed with the weak and the infirm." (Counter at approximately **33:40-35:19**.)

Question

What do you think of Scrooge's remark? Is there some truth in it? What role do you think this attitude played in his becoming a bitter man?

Could you say that you share this opinion of the world to some degree? Why or why not?

Cut 4

Scrooge meets the Ghost of Christmas Present. He shows that joy is unfamiliar to him.
"I am too old and beyond hope. . . . " (Counter at approximately **48:49-51:15**.)

Question

Is anyone too old and beyond hope?

Cut 5

Scrooge sees people in the poorhouse singing on Christmas. (Counter at approximately **51:15-52:06**.)

Question

How could people be joyful and singing when their lives are so bad?
If joy doesn't come from having good things or having an easy life, where does it come from?

Cut 6

Scrooge has awakened from the dream and discovers joy. He tells the boy to buy the prize turkey which he plans to give to his employee, Bob Cratchit.
"Bells, bells. What a beautiful morning."
"Intelligent boy. Remarkable boy." (Counter at approximately **1:17:28-1:18:53**.)

Questions

Comment on Scrooge's joy. How do you know he's not having a manic episode?
What would Scrooge have said of the boy before his transformation? How does the experience of joy change the way he sees others? The world?
Scrooge is joyful over ordinary things (bells, the boy). Why?

Cut 7

Scrooge goes to his nephew's house for Christmas. He is hesitant to go in at first and feels awkward about asking if he can stay for dinner. He also apologizes to his nephew's wife. (Counter at approximately **1:19:24-1:22:13**.)

Questions

Notice how awkward it is for Scrooge to reintegrate himself with others. Have you ever experienced this? Do you sometimes feel awkward around people who are having a good time? Why?

IT'S A WONDERFUL LIFE

Cut 1

George Bailey acknowledges that he wants to live again. He is filled with joy. You see how much he appreciates everything— his children, his house, even the people who came to arrest him. His wife is also privileged to experience joy. (Counter at approximately **2:04:30-end of movie**.)

Discussion

Just comment on the scene. Again, it's possible that bipolar people may say that George Bailey is having a manic episode. Be prepared to help them distinguish a manic episode from a genuine experience of joy.

Homework

Are you willing to put joy in your life this holiday season? What would you be willing to experience as joyful?

Chapter 12

Affective Issues

Some people have little access to their feelings. This may be partly due to the psychiatric illness itself, such as the flat affect often seen in schizophrenics. It may be due to a lack of socialization, or to dynamic conflicts. It also may be due to a combination of these factors. Groups designed to help people get in touch with their feelings, therefore, may be useful.

Nothing More Than Feelings is a group designed for this purpose. In addition to helping people identify their feelings, it touches on key issues that patients may have to deal with, such as the insensitivity of others in the community toward the psychiatrically ill, and the feelings one might have in a first interview with a new mental health worker.

Patients may be able to identify with Conrad, the protagonist of the film that is used (*Ordinary People*), who was suicidally depressed and cannot get over the death of his brother in a boating accident. This is a double-edged sword. It may be helpful that the protagonist has psychiatric problems just like the patients. On the other hand, some patients may become unduly anxious about the discussion of suicide. With this film, as well as all films that you use, you will need to judge whether or not it is appropriate for your group. The perfect film for one group of psychiatric patients might be totally inappropriate for the next group.

For example, I once planned to use clips from the film *A Home of Our Own* for a group. On the day that the group was scheduled, a new patient arrived who had survived a major explosion that occurred at her apartment complex, leaving her homeless. The group was swiftly canceled and another put in its place. Usually, I am not a risk-taker in this regard. I do recall one time, however, when the group consisted of high-functioning patients, some of whom had been suicidal in the past, who needed to be instilled with a sense of possibility. I considered showing the film *My Left Foot.* The film is full of difficult scenes in which there are family fights, the protagonist becomes suicidal, and more. I thought for a long time about whether or not to show it. I considered carefully each person who was in the program and how each individual would experience various parts of the film. In the end, I decided to take a gamble. I stayed in the room the entire time. There were three or four times when I cringed inside, thinking that I must have been crazy to show the film. The discussion that ensued, however, was very positive. The film woke people up and the discussion infused them with a different sense of themselves. It was a gamble that turned out well.

Remember to always preview any film you show. I once made the mistake of showing a film that was highly recommended by someone in the mental health center. The person swore to me that the movie included no scenes that might be traumatic for the patients. In reality, there were traumatic scenes of family violence and, at one point, a date rape. My first instinct was to shoot the person who recommended the film; however, it was really my fault for not previewing it. I had to clean up the mess in group therapy. Don't learn the hard way.

Mania and Joy combines a brainstorming exercise with a movie clip. One bipolar patient who participated in this group realized that he was not with everyone else in the world during manic episodes, as he had fancied, but rather that he was alone in his own world. Weeks later when he was saying good-bye on his last day, he pointed to this revelation as a turning point in his relationship with his illness. It was this revelation that caused him to give up the desire to be manic.

The Self-Expression Game is a therapeutic game that helps people to become more expressive. The game is best played with higher-functioning patients who can think abstractly and have some frustration tolerance. I had a funny experience the first time I ran this game. One of the clues I used to get people to a pay phone in the hall was, "It's the next best thing to being there." I thought it was obvious. No one got the clue. When I later explained that it had been a slogan for an advertisement, no one remembered the advertisement. Finally someone said, "Oh, yeah! But that was a *long* time ago!"

NOTHING MORE THAN FEELINGS

Introduction of Theme

Opening Questions

This group is about exploring our feelings as well as our reluctance to experience our feelings. Why do you think that people are often reluctant to acknowledge their feelings?

Are you reluctant to feel your feelings? If so, why?

Introduction of Movie

We will use the movie *Ordinary People* for this group. This movie involves an adolescent named Conrad and his parents. Conrad's older brother died earlier in a boating accident. Conrad never got over this. At one point, he attempted suicide. The movie is about his relationship with his parents, his peers, and his psychiatrist.

Movie Cuts and Questions

ORDINARY PEOPLE

Cut 1

Conrad pretends that he is studying in bed when he is really anxious and unable to sleep. He hides this from his father. (Counter at approximately **5:30-7:14**.)

Questions

From whom do you hide your problems? From whom do you hide your feelings? Why?

Cut 2

The mother is cold toward her son. The father is worried and faking it with his son. (Counter at approximately **7:36-10:15**.)

Questions

What do you think is going on with Conrad's mother? How do you think the rest of the family is affected by her coldness? Can you relate to anyone in this scene?

Cut 3

> Conrad talks to himself in the elevator to rehearse what he will say when he sees the psychiatrist. (Counter at approximately **16:01-16:51**.)

Questions

Isn't it a relief to know that we all talk to ourselves? Why do you think we do that?

Why do you think Conrad is nervous about seeing the psychiatrist? Can you relate?

Cut 4

> This is Conrad's first visit with the psychiatrist. It's awkward. Conrad resents the questions. (Counter at approximately **16:51-21:13**.)

Discussion

Give patients full permission to discuss how they feel about being asked so many questions by staff during evaluations, being asked the same questions by various people, being asked embarrassing questions, etc.

Cut 5

> The coach asks insensitive questions and makes inappropriate remarks. (Counter at approximately **22:25-23:37**.)

Discussion

Encourage people to discuss their feelings about others' insensitivity regarding their psychiatric problems.

Cut 6

Mother and Conrad bump into each other in Brett's room. They talk surface talk—no real issues. (Counter at approximately **26:30-29:12**.)

Questions

What would these two have discussed if they had been more open? What might they have said to one another? Why do you think they avoided the real issues?

Have you ever avoided talking about real issues with someone? Why?

Cut 7

Conrad's father and mother are at a party. His father tells a friend that Conrad is seeing a psychiatrist. His mother later gets upset, stating that this is "family business." (Counter at approximately **32:00-33:35**.)

Questions

What do you think of what Conrad's father did? Of his mother's position?

Why do you think that discussing psychiatric issues is so taboo? What are people afraid of? How do you feel about discussing psychiatric issues with nonpatients?

Cut 8

Conrad: "50 bucks an hour. Can't you decide if I should have a pill or not, I mean, you're a doctor! I'm supposed to feel better, right?"

Dr. B: "Not necessarily." (Counter at approximately **33:35-36:15**.)

Discussion

Have patients discuss this. Relate this to any myths they have that medication will solve all their problems.

Cut 9

The psychiatrist makes Conrad angry.

Conrad: "It takes too much energy to get mad."

Dr. B: "You know how much energy it takes to hold it back?"

Conrad: "When I let myself feel, all I feel is lousy."

Dr. B: "A little advice about feeling, kiddo. Don't expect it always to tickle." (Counter at approximately **53:30-55:51**.)

Discussion

Elicit comments about this scene. Focus on people's tendencies to repress anger, if that is appropriate.

Cut 10

This is a precious and funny scene of Conrad awkwardly asking his friend for a date. Besides helping people to discuss their awkwardness about dating, it provides some levity in a heavy group. (Counter at approximately **1:01:58-1:05:00**.)

Questions

How do you feel about asking others out for a date? About dating? About romance and sexuality in general?

Cut 11

Conrad feels very guilty about trying to kill himself and believes that he can't be forgiven. (Counter at approximately **1:09:50-1:11:49**.)

Questions

Have you forgiven yourself for the mistakes you made in your life? Talk about the role that guilt plays in your life.

Cut 12

This is the big scene in the movie where Conrad has the break-through.

> Conrad realizes that he feels guilty because he stayed with the boat when his brother was drowning.
> Conrad: "I'm scared."
> Dr. B: "Feelings are scary. And sometimes they're painful. And if you can't feel pain then you're not going to feel anything else either." (Counter at approximately **1:39:01-1:46:21**.)

Questions

What do you think about what the psychiatrist said?

We all feel guilty about things. What power are you allowing guilt to have over your life? What's the best way to handle guilt?

Homework

Write a brief assessment of your relationship with your feelings. How much do you allow yourself to feel? What do you allow yourself to feel? What feelings are not allowed? Why?

MANIA AND JOY

(Combination movie group and exercise group)

Introductory Comments

People with bipolar illness are often afraid to have feelings. One feeling they are afraid of is happiness. This is because they can't distinguish it from mania. Often patients say that "I'm afraid to feel happy because I'm afraid it means I'm getting sick." This is particularly true about strong feelings such as extreme sadness, even if it's appropriate, such as during a funeral.

Introduction of Movie

One way to illustrate this difficulty is demonstrated in the movie *It's a Wonderful Life.* This is the story of George Bailey, a very kind man who often sacrifices his own desires to meet others' needs. When a tragic event occurs concerning his place of business, he has the urge to commit suicide. An angel rescues him from this desire by showing him what a difference his life makes to others. Toward the end of the movie, George has an entirely different experience of his life. Let's see what it is.

Movie Cut and Questions

IT'S A WONDERFUL LIFE

Cut 1

In this scene, George is elated because he is back to reality where people know who he is. He is deeply joyful about his home, his children, and all of his life. (Counter at approximately **2:04:30-end of movie**.)

Questions

Is George having a manic episode or is he joyful? How do you know?

Exercise

Have patients make two lists side by side on the board. One list will include the characteristics of mania while the opposite will include the characteristics of happiness or joy. Here are some examples from a group that I conducted:

MANIA	HAPPINESS/JOY
Out of control	In control
Based on misperceptions; delusions	Grounded in reality
Accompanied by depression	Depression not present
Not lasting	Can be lasting—no inherent "crash"
Can't be shared or understood	Can be shared
Racing thoughts present	No racing thoughts
Personality change	Stable personality
Poor decisions that hurt self and/or others	Decision-making ability intact

Have patients generate their own list. These items might be included by you if any of them are missed.

Next have patients generate a list of occasions in which it would be perfectly natural for someone to be happy. This also can be done on the board.

Finish with a general discussion about the impact that this will have on their lives.

SELF-EXPRESSION GAME

Preparation

This group takes a lot of time to prepare but it is well worth it with the right group of patients. The preparation consists of preparing the clues.

The game is a treasure hunt for which clues have been placed all over the building. On each clue is also written an instruction that involves self-expression, such as singing, telling a story, joking, etc.

First you must come up with seven places in the building where you can hide clues and, if desired, small goodies like gum or pieces of candy (this is optional). Make sure to use places where other patients and professionals will not be unduly disturbed by the goings-on of the game.

Next you will prepare the clues. (See page 210 for sample clues). Let us imagine that you will have ten patients. The patients will be working in pairs, meaning that you will have five pairs of patients. These pairs will be labeled A through E. Since you will have eight clues, the clues will be labeled 1 through 8. This means the clues will be labeled as follows: A-1, A-2, A-3, etc. to A-8, B-1, B-2, etc. to B-8, etc., corresponding to the patient labels. Label the top left corner of the pieces of paper. You may also label the backs of the clues.

Next you should write the self-expression instructions. Make up eight things that they can do such as:

- Sing the first verse of your favorite song.
- Make up a four-line poem that begins "Roses are red, violets are blue. . . . "
- Tell a fictional short story.
- Tell a nonfictional short story from your life.
- Tell a joke.
- Tell your partner one thing that you like about him/her.
- Play charades.
- Imitate your favorite movie star.

One each of the eight instructions should be written on the top half of each of the eight pages. Place a solid line in the middle of the page dividing the top and bottom halves of the page (See Figure 12.1).

FIGURE 12.1

A-1

Sing the first verse of your favorite song.

People can come here when they're thirsty but they can't drink for free!

The clues can be handwritten.

The bottom halves of the pages will give the clues about where the next clue is hidden. Make the challenges minimal. When I first practiced this game, I made the mistake of making the clues too hard, which frustrated the entire group. Keep in mind that the clues may seem too easy to you because you know the answers. If anything, however, err on the side of making the clues too easy. Here are some examples:

1. People can come here when they are thirsty but they can't drink for free. (Soda machine)
2. This place has seen many a winner—and many a loser. (Gym)
3. This isn't a good place to work for people who can't stand the sight of blood. (Lab)
4. Many a magazine is read here. (Waiting room)
5. This place is very popular at noon. (Cafeteria)
6. This place gives you a way to get in touch with people when you can't actually see them. Bring your change! (Pay phone)
7. You'll see more pills in this place than anywhere else. (Pharmacy)
8. This is a very private place and one where men and women do not meet. (Bathroom)

The last thing to do is to hide the clues. Again, don't do too good a job. I made that mistake, too. I had patients who found the right place but then couldn't find the clue. (In this instance, they got to the inpatient unit but didn't think to look under the large mat where I placed the clues. I had to go up with them and give them more clues verbally.)

Clue #1 is not hidden (you will hand that to the patients). All the clue #2s are hidden together, all the clue #3s, etc. Clues A2, B2, C2, D2 and E2 all say the same thing and are hidden in one place together, such as the gym. Clues A3, B3, C3, etc., all say the same thing and are hidden in a same place, such as the lab, and so on down to the last clues.

Activity

The first clue is handed to the patients in the day room. The bottom half directs them to clue #2. That means that the pair of patients labeled "A" receive clue A1. They must find A2, A3, etc.

Emphasize that they must do the self-expression portion, not skip it. Some of them will skip it anyway. This will be part of the discussion.

Be sure that you stay in one place (the day room would be good) so that patients can come to you for help when they get stuck.

Discussion

Did you have fun? If not, why not? Did you allow yourself to let go?

Which self-expression instructions did you skip or do halfheartedly? Why?

How well did you and your partner work together? Did one of you take the lead? How did you feel about this?

Chapter 13

About Exercise

Exercise can be difficult to justify in a day hospital program because it appears to be unrelated to the immediate psychiatric need. Since I am not an expert on physiology or physical fitness, I cannot comment extensively on the relationship between the mind and body. There are writers who comment extensively on this matter. Mainstream medicine is examining this more closely as well.

What we can consider are some of the psychiatric components of the exercise group. More often than not, exercise groups consist of some kind of team sport such as badminton, volleyball, softball, basketball, etc. Viewed from the standpoint of interaction, many psychiatric issues can be addressed inside of a sports event.

Amotivation	Use the group to improve the person's motivation to play and to win.
Anhedonia	How much pleasure does the person receive from therapeutic recreation? How might s/he transfer this into his or her daily life setting?
Anxiety	How anxious is the patient about the game? How comfortable is the patient with taking risks?
Dependency	Does this person exhibit any autonomy on the playing field? Does s/he manipulate others into taking responsibility for him/her during the game? Use the game to improve autonomy.
Dysphoria, blunted or flat affect	Does the person's affect brighten during the game?

Inappropriate affect	Does the person respond appropriately to the events of the game—disappointment when striking out, happy with home run, etc.?
Integrity	This is particularly problematic for those recovering from addiction and those with certain Axis II diagnoses, such as antisocial personality disorder and borderline personality disorder. Discourage cheating and insist on integrity on the playing field.
Internal preoccupation	Is the person attentive to the situation or lost in his or her own world? Use the group to keep him or her engaged in life.
Isolation	How much does this person interact with others? Use the group to improve interaction.
Poor interpersonal skills	Is this person a team player? How does s/he handle winning and losing?
Poor judgment	What kind of judgment is used in making strategic decisions? Use the group to help the patient think through decisions more appropriately.
Poor self-esteem	Does the patient exhibit self-confidence on the playing field? Does s/he berate him/herself for mistakes and/or acknowledge successes?
Psychosis	What is the patient's interpretation of the events surrounding him/her? Improve reality testing.

I recommend setting a psychiatric exercise goal for each patient and charting their progress during the course of their stays in the day hospital. By "charting their progress" I mean to make their progress with the goals the content of the progress notes about exercise. Incidental notes about physical benefits could be added if desired.

Chapter 14

Versatility

This chapter focuses on versatility—taking what is already there and adapting it to meet your needs. Remember my earlier advice that one should look at everything as potential material for the day hospital. One of the things you can do is to go to the local toy store and look at the games. Might these games be adapted to meet your needs? Again, you want the games to serve your therapeutic purposes. You don't want to invent erroneous clinical goals to fit the game that you have. It doesn't hurt, however, to just look over the games and see what creative thoughts they inspire.

Old Maid with a Twist didn't come to me while I was playing Old Maid (I think I was seven the last time I played it). It was just one of those ideas that plunked itself into my mind uninvited. Patients have had a lot of fun with it. Just remember to collect all the cards when the game is over or else you'll have more than one "old maid."

A few other common games that can be adapted to meet therapeutic needs are also discussed. I've used the Monopoly idea at times when the group had done a lot of heavy-duty clinical work and needed a break. You'd be surprised why people buy property—"because I like the color green," "because I always buy this property," etc. The checkers idea was used once with a patient who refused to obey day hospital rules. It proved an excellent avenue through which we could explore his relationship with rules.

I also discuss the use of two games from the book *Games Trainers Play* by Edward Scannell and John W. Newstrom. I specifically focus on the way the games were adapted to meet the needs of the psychiatric patients.

The last group discussed in this chapter is Making Sense of Our Senses, a group I designed to help patients explore healthier ways to experience pleasure. Not only did the patients enjoy the sensual aspects of the exercise, it also provided a forum for trust. They had to close their eyes and trust that what I asked them to smell or feel would not be repulsive. They sometimes struggled with this but eventually allowed my soft voice and gentle encouragement to enroll them in a little trust.

OLD MAID WITH A TWIST

Preparation

Use index cards to prepare a "playing deck." Choose a theme such as conflict resolution on the job.

Construct a number of scenarios relating to your theme to use for role-play. For example, using the theme of "conflict resolution on the job," the following scenarios might be constructed: Your boss asks you out for a date, your co-worker is drinking on the job, your immediate supervisor is making you do his work, your boss is angry with you and you don't know why.

Write these scenarios on the index cards. Write a duplicate for all except one of the scenarios.

Activity

Shuffle the "deck" thoroughly and deal the cards to the patients. Have a participant read one card. Whoever has the other card with that theme will be this person's partner in role-playing the situation. Both will come to the front of the room and do the role-play with coaching. At the end of the game, one person will be left with a card that has a theme and has no match. That person is the "old maid"!

Discussion

Discussion should be inherent in the role-play. Treat it like an assertiveness-training group.

GAMES MADE THERAPEUTIC

Preparation

Have the appropriate board game handy. Make sure you have more than one copy of the game if you have many people.

Activity

Monopoly

Have patients play Monopoly according to the rules. Whenever they have the opportunity to buy a piece of property, they should end their turn by telling the group *why* they decided to buy or not to buy. The same is true for other decisions in the game such as whether or not to pay to get out of jail. No explanation is needed for moves they are forced to make such as going to jail when they get the "go to jail" card.

Checkers

This can be made into a game of invention. Begin with traditional checkers. Then ask the patients to come up with at least one other way to play a game with a board, squares, and black and red pieces. They make up the rules. They should then play a game according to their own rules.

Example: Instead of jumping over your opponent's pieces to capture them, you can land on top of your opponent's pieces. Your opponent is forced to stay in that place until you move. You get an extra turn when you land on your opponent.

Hangman

Play hangman according to the rules with the stipulation that the words chosen must relate to a theme of your choice. The theme could be relapse prevention, medicine, addiction recovery, etc.

Charades

Essentially the same as above. Play charades according to the rules except that the words or phrases must relate to a theme of your choice.

BALLOON FRANTIC: ADAPTING THERAPEUTIC GAMES

Balloon Frantic is a therapeutic game found in the book titled *Games Trainers Play* by Scannell and Newstrom. Participants blow up balloons. The object of the game is to keep the balloons in the air for as long as possible. They are allowed to use any body part to accomplish this goal.

How can this game be made therapeutic for a psychiatric population? People who are impulsive can be encouraged to play mindfully and slowly. Instead of running all over the room while hitting the balloons hard, making it difficult to keep them in the air, they can hit the balloons softly and keep them in one area. People who are anhedonic or lack motivation due to the negative symptoms of schizophrenia can be encouraged to be more active. They should hit the balloons harder and have to move a little more. People who are narcissistic should be encouraged to develop a team strategy for keeping the balloons in the air. Their focus will be to keep the best interest of the entire team in mind as they play.

Extremely low-functioning individuals, such as someone with Alzheimer's disease, might be flanked by three people, one on either side and one in back. Those support people would be responsible for hitting the balloons back toward the patient when they start to go out of bounds. For example, you might have two such patients up front, each of them flanked by three other patients. They can hit the balloons back and forth with help from those on the side. This gives them an opportunity to succeed, something they may rarely experience. It gives the others an opportunity to support someone as well.

People who are depressed or too restricted in their affect should be encouraged to take risks and have fun. You know you've hit pay dirt when someone who never cracks a smile starts giggling. When the activity is over, have this person process what it feels like to let go and laugh.

BIRTHDAY WALL: ADAPTING THERAPEUTIC GAMES

Another game found in *Games Trainers Play* is the Birthday Wall. In this game, players line up on a piece of paper or line. With eyes closed, they must order themselves according to birthdays. Other variations include ordering themselves according to shoe size or height. If anyone steps off the paper or the line, all must go back to their original places and begin the process again.

This game can be made therapeutic for a psychiatric population in various ways. First play the game with no instructions other than the ones outlined above. Notice who takes the leadership role and who doesn't. Invariably there will be people who do nothing—who allow others to push them to their proper place and offer nothing more to the group process. Some of those people may be capable of doing more. Process the first game, taking note of people's performance with regard to this dynamic. Then ask the more passive people to lead. You can ask specific people to lead through parts of the exercise. Several things may be accomplished this way: someone who lacks self-confidence can have an experience of being a successful leader; someone who rarely talks may be forced to talk; someone who is chronically dependent on others may be forced to assume some autonomy. At the same time, impulsive and intrusive people will be encouraged to follow rather than lead. People who have a hard time listening to instructions should be followers. Just listening should be their goal.

As always, the game should end with discussion to relate the events of the game to the patients' day-to-day lives.

MAKING SENSE OF OUR SENSES

Preparation

You will need five groups of items. Be sure to keep the five groups separate. Two items per group will suffice.

Group #1: Sense of Smell

Fragrant flower, cinnamon, almond extract, shampoo, soap, suntan lotion, lemon or orange, perfume or cologne, potpourri.

Group #2: Sense of Touch

Fur coat, fan, feather, plant with "furry" leaves.

Group #3: Sense of Sound

Tapes of whales, rain in forest, ocean waves.

Group #4: Sense of Sight

Pretty flower or plant, pretty scarf, pictures, soft light.

Group #5: Sense of Taste

Aspartame (any brand), cooked red Idaho potato, grapes (sweet).

Cover each group with a cloth or large piece of white paper. Also, hang five sheets of large, white paper on the wall.

Opening Questions

1. How many of you have difficulty enjoying anything most of the time?

   Note: This can lead to a discussion about anhedonia as a component of depression, if appropriate.

2. How many of you find that the ways you pursue pleasure are sometimes not good for you? The following list of possibilities might help you in answering this question: Overeating, smoking, illicit drug use, abuse of prescription drugs such as major tranquilizers, excessive or inappropriate sex, excessive exercise. (This is not an exhaustive list.)

   If desired, take some time to discuss this.

3. How many of you find that you are relatively unaware of the sounds around you, the taste of your food, etc.? Do you really "take time to smell the flowers"? Or are you barely aware of the flowers?

Activity

Smell

Instruct the patients to close their eyes. Assure them that you will not do anything to frighten or startle them. Explain that you will walk up to each one of them with something for them to smell. They are to try to guess what the scent is. They are not to say anything, however, so others can guess as well.

As you approach each patient, call her or his name softly so s/he is not startled. Put the item close to her or his nose and allow the person to sniff. You can ask, "OK?" to make sure the patient smelled it. Look at each person's eyes to see if they look tense. Reassure them if closing their eyes appears to be threatening.

Once you are through, ask the patients to open their eyes and guess the scent.

Repeat this entire process with the second scent you chose.

Touch

Have patients close their eyes again. This time have them touch the fur coat or other material. They should again try to guess what it is without saying anything out loud. As you approach each person, gently take one hand and put it on the item. If you are concerned that this will startle someone or that trust, in the area of touch, is a major issue, verbally instruct the patient to reach out and touch the item. Bring the item to the outstretched hand.

Again have patients open their eyes and guess the item. Do this again with a second item, perhaps the leaf of a plant that feels good to the touch (all stimuli should be pleasant to the senses).

Sound

Now ask patients to close their eyes and listen to the tapes. Play each of the two tapes for a few minutes and then briefly discuss.

Sight

This part will obviously entail no guessing. You can hold up the scarf or one or two of the pictures. Discuss their esthetic value. You can put on the soft light and discuss the role of lighting in emotions—how a soft light might be calming, sexy, etc.

Taste

This also will not be an "eyes closed" exercise. Put a little bit of aspartame in each person's hand. Have each one taste it and really notice how sweet it is. Then give each patient a piece of the cooked potato. Instruct them to eat it slowly, noticing the taste of a potato. Ask them to describe it afterward. Discuss our propensity for putting butter, sour cream, salt and pepper, etc., on the potato instead of just tasting the potato. A potato by itself has approximately 25 carbohydrates and contains no fat. A potato with butter or sour cream is quite fattening.

Exercise

Have five patients volunteer to be writers. Using magic markers, each will be assigned to one of the large pieces of paper on the wall and one of the senses.

The entire group is to call out ways that each of these senses can be experienced or enjoyed in a way that is healthy and inexpensive. These ways are to be written on the sheets. For example, one might enjoy the sense of hearing by having windchimes, listening to a cat's purr, or listening to the wind.

Final Question

What is the difference between being sensual and being hedonistic?

Chapter 15

Ending the Day

We talked about ways to begin the day in the beginning of the book. What would be some ways to end the day?

One might end the day with the question, "What did you learn today?" This helps people to summarize their day and to create some value from it. The only unacceptable answers are "I don't know" and "nothing." If the patient can't identify what s/he learned, the therapist can point to some accomplishment and frame it in terms of learning. ("I noticed that you stayed in the room all day without leaving to pace in the hallway.")

If Five-Day Project Creation goals are up on the wall, you might have patients check off whatever goals they achieved over the preceding twenty-four hours. This allows them to see progress throughout the week (or lack of progress, which might motivate them).

Another way to end the day is with something inspirational such as a song, poem, or saying.

Of course it is important to make sure that all logistics have been handled. This would include making sure that patients have their medication and that the day room and kitchen areas are cleaned. I think it is important for patients to take responsibility for that. It is *their* day program. *They* should clean out the coffee pot and put on the coffee in the morning. *They* should put away the markers and clean out the sink.

It is important to find out who plans to be out the next day in order to ensure that they have enough medication to cover them until they return. The end of the day is also a good time to make a mental check of who you might have concerns about sending home. Make sure such people were evaluated by the psychiatrist before you let them go. It is important that you control when people leave so that you don't discover that people who must see the psychiatrist or haven't received their meds have slipped out the door.

I always feel exhausted after the patients leave. The lack of noise stands out. I suddenly give myself permission to let go, to be tired. It's a good idea to mentally review your own accomplishments with the group over the course of the day, to have a little bit of closure for yourself before diving into those progress notes, returning phone calls, etc. Congratulate yourself on a job well done.

Bibliography

Alonso, Anne and Swiller, Hillel (Eds.). (1993). *Group therapy in clinical practice.* Washington, DC: American Psychiatric Press, Inc.

American Psychiatric Association (1994). *Diagnostic and statistical manual of mental disorders,* Fourth Edition. Washington, DC: Author.

Beck, Aaron T. (1985). *Anxiety disorders and phobias: A cognitive perspective.* New York: Basic Books.

Beck, Aaron T., Rush, J., Shaw, B., and Emery, G. (1979). *Cognitive therapy of depression.* New York: The Guilford Press, 1979.

Bourne, Edmund J. (1990). *The anxiety and phobia workbook.* Oakland, CA: New Harbinger Publications, Inc.

Brabender, Virginia and Fallon, April (1993). *Models of inpatient group psychotherapy.* Washington, DC: American Psychological Association.

Budman, Simon H. and Gurman, Alan S. (1988). *Theory and practice of brief therapy.* New York: The Guilford Press.

Copeland, Mary Ellen (1992). *The depression workbook.* Oakland, CA: New Harbinger Publications, Inc.

Davis, Martha, Eshelman, Elizabeth Robbins, and McKay, Matthew (1988). *The relaxation and stress reduction workbook.* Oakland, CA: New Harbinger Publications, Inc.

Erikson, Erik H. (1980). *Identity and the life cycle.* New York: W.W. Norton.

Erikson, Erik H. (1985). *Childhood and society.* New York: W.W. Norton.

Evans, Gloria Jay (1977). *The wall.* Waco, TX: Word Books.

Freud, S. (1973). *Abstracts of the standard edition of the complete psychological works.* New York: International University Press.

Friedman, William H. (1994). *How to do groups.* Northvale, NJ: Jason Aronson, Inc.

Goldberg, Carl and Goldberg, Merle Cantor (1973). *The human circle: An existential approach to the new group therapies.* Chicago: Nelson Hall Co.

Horney, Karen (1985). *Collected works of Karen Horney.* New York: W.W. Norton.

Kaplan, Harold and Saddock, Benjamin (Eds.). (1993). *Comprehensive group psychotherapy.* Third Edition. Baltimore: Williams and Wilkins.

Kaplan, Kathy L. (1988). *Directive group therapy.* Thorofare, NJ: Slack Inc.

Kernberg, Otto (1985). *Borderline conditions and pathological narcissism.* Northvale, NJ: Jason Aronson.

Kernberg, Otto (1986) (c. 1984). *Object relations theory and clinical psychoanalysis.* Northvale, NJ: Jason Aronson.

Lewis, C.S. (1953). *The silver chair.* New York: Macmillan Publishing Company.

Mahler, Margaret S. (1975). *The psychological birth of the human infant: Symbiosis and individuation.* New York: Basic Books.

Mahler, Margaret S. (1979). *The selected papers of Margaret S. Mahler, MD.* New York: Jason Aronson, 1979.

Mandino, Og. *The God memorandum.* Hollywood, FL: Lifetime Books.

May, Rollo (1983). *The discovery of being: Writings in existential psychology.* First Edition. New York: W.W. Norton.

Minuchin, Salvador (1974). *Families and family therapy.* Cambridge, MA: Harvard University Press.

Rice, Cecil A. and Rutan, J. Scott (1987). *Inpatient group psychotherapy: A psychodynamic perspective.* New York: Macmillan Publishing Co.

Rutan, J. Scott and Stone, Walter N. (1993). *Psychodynamic group psychotherapy.* Second Edition. New York: The Guilford Press.

Scannell, Edward and Newstrom, John W. (1980). *Games trainers play.* New York: McGraw-Hill, Inc.

Sullivan, Harry S. (1953). *The interpersonal theory of psychiatry.* New York: W.W. Norton.

Sullivan, Harry S. (1965) (c. 1940-64). *Collected works.* New York: W.W. Norton.

Yalom, Irvin D. (1980). *Existential psychotherapy.* New York: Basic Books.

Yalom, Irvin D. (1983). *Inpatient group psychotherapy.* New York: Basic Books, Inc.

Yalom, Irvin D. (1983). *The theory and practice of group psychotherapy.* New York: Basic Books.

Index

Order Your Own Copy of
This Important Book for Your Personal Library!

A GUIDE TO CREATIVE GROUP PROGRAMMING IN THE PSYCHIATRIC DAY HOSPITAL

_____ in hardbound at $39.95 (ISBN: 0-7890-0406-2)

COST OF BOOKS _____

OUTSIDE USA/CANADA/
MEXICO: ADD 20% _____

POSTAGE & HANDLING _____
(US: $3.00 for first book & $1.25
for each additional book)
Outside US: $4.75 for first book
& $1.75 for each additional book)

SUBTOTAL _____

IN CANADA: ADD 7% GST _____

STATE TAX _____
(NY, OH & MN residents, please
add appropriate local sales tax)

FINAL TOTAL _____
(If paying in Canadian funds,
convert using the current
exchange rate. UNESCO
coupons welcome.)

☐ **BILL ME LATER:** ($5 service charge will be added)
(Bill-me option is good on US/Canada/Mexico orders only;
not good to jobbers, wholesalers, or subscription agencies.)

☐ Check here if billing address is different from
shipping address and attach purchase order and
billing address information.

Signature _____

☐ **PAYMENT ENCLOSED: $** _____

☐ **PLEASE CHARGE TO MY CREDIT CARD.**

☐ Visa ☐ MasterCard ☐ AmEx ☐ Discover

Account # _____

Exp. Date _____

Signature _____

Prices in US dollars and subject to change without notice.

NAME _____

INSTITUTION _____

ADDRESS _____

CITY _____

STATE/ZIP _____

COUNTRY _____ COUNTY (NY residents only) _____

TEL _____ FAX _____

E-MAIL_____
May we use your e-mail address for confirmations and other types of information? ☐ Yes ☐ No

Order From Your Local Bookstore or Directly From
The Haworth Press, Inc.
10 Alice Street, Binghamton, New York 13904-1580 • USA
TELEPHONE: 1-800-HAWORTH (1-800-429-6784) / Outside US/Canada: (607) 722-5857
FAX: 1-800-895-0582 / Outside US/Canada: (607) 772-6362
E-mail: getinfo@haworth.com
PLEASE PHOTOCOPY THIS FORM FOR YOUR PERSONAL USE.

BOF96

BELMONT UNIVERSITY LIBRARY